"This book tells what my cancer patients need to know to make choices about doctors and treatments; detailed and precise, this is a very honest book— hopeful and realistic at the same time. I will recommend it to my cancer patients and their families."

Richard Adair, M.D., F.A.C.P.
Clinical Assistant Professor of Medicine
University of Minnesota School of Medicine

"With any technical subject, the specialist must communicate. Dr. Anku does this admirably and compassionately. This book helps focus on the methods available in the medical arsenal for cancer treatment without sacrificing the humanity of either physician or patient. It emphasizes not just what is medically possible, but what is medically possible in the context of quality of living, rather than just living."

Mrs. Theresa F. Mihelich
Strongsville, Ohio

"This book is a compassionate and hopeful presentation of an emotionally charged subject. The scientific, factual information is presented in simple, readable language that is easily understood by the layperson. The author's expertise, experience and humanism are evident throughout this book. It should be read by everyone concerned with cancer."

Evans Z. Fiakpui, M.S., M.D., F.A.C.O.G.
Assistant Professor, University of Chicago Lying-in Hospital
Department of Obstetrics and Gynecology

"Having undergone chemotherapy twice as well as radiation therapy, I am most impressed with this book. The style is down-to-earth and the text so clearly stated that it is very easy for the lay person to understand. As a leader of a Cancer Therapy Cope Group, I look forward to sharing this book and its inspirational message with our group members and friends. It indeed gives reason for hope, for coping with the pain and anxiety in simple, honest terms."

Mary Jane Hase Smith
Orlando, Florida

"Dr. Anku outlines the philosophy of modern cancer treatment in great detail. The tone of the text is quite optimistic and emphasizes several important concepts in modern oncology. The book will be of great interest to the patient and will be extremely useful for the relatives of persons undergoing cancer treatment."

John E. Feldmann, M.D.
Medical Oncologist
Mobile, Alabama

"An admirable job of providing patients and their families a clearly written agenda for dealing with cancer. The book conveys the importance of and the power of positive thinking, and should help prevent the crippling effects of despair, confusion, fear, and lack of understanding."

Ted Doering, M.D.
Pediatric Oncologist
President, Western Reserve Childrens
Cancer Research Foundation

"Dr. Anku has achieved the goal of helping cancer victims and their families understand their disease and the different types of treatment along with side effects and consequences of the treatment. This book will take away a lot of anxiety about cancer."

Vishwa M. Sharan, M.D.
Assistant Professor in Radiology
Case Western Reserve University

"Dr. Anku has taken a very complicated subject and written a book which can be easily understood by everyone. He presents a very positive approach to a very serious condition, cancer. Those who read the book can learn a great deal from it, whether they are dealing with cancer personally or just want to become better informed on the subject."

Russell F. Catanese, Executive Director
American Cancer Society, Cuyahoga County Unit

"*What to Know About the Treatment of Cancer* is the first book to give us lay people a greatly needed understanding of one of the most feared health hazards of our time. It emphasizes the great importance of early detection and proper treatment, which often makes the difference between life and death. The stress and concern of having or maybe having cancer one day can only be resolved by educating oneself on the subject. This book successfully does that. It should be made available in every library of our educational system."

Leonard and Corrie Llewellyn
Marco Beach, Florida
(Mr. Llewellyn is a former member of the board of trustees of Naples Community Hospital; his wife has been a leader in American Cancer Society programs in Southwest Florida.)

WHAT
TO KNOW
ABOUT THE
TREATMENT
OF CANCER

VINCENT ANKU, M.D.

MADRONA PUBLISHERS   SEATTLE   1984

Dedicated to Dr. Lee Tressel

Published by
Madrona Publishers, Inc.
P.O. Box 22667
Seattle, Washington 98122

10 9 8 7 6 5 4 3 2

Library of Congress Cataloging in Publication Data

Anku, Vincent, 1940–
    What to know about the treatment of cancer.

    Bibliography: p.
    Includes index.
    1. Cancer—Chemotherapy. 2. Antineoplastic agents.
3. Oncology—Popular works. I. Title. [DNLM:
1. Neoplasms—drug therapy—popular works.   QZ 201 A611w]
RC271.C5A63   1984   616.99'406   84-20148
ISBN 0–88089–002–9

Foreword

Developments in the therapy of cancer have been burgeoning at such a rapid rate that the public, and often physicians themselves, have become bewildered and confused over what has been done and can be done to treat this often frightening, overwhelming malady. For many years, there has been an obvious need for an up-to-date, sensible publication on cancer and its treatment.

What to Know About the Treatment of Cancer is the answer to this need. Written by a highly qualified oncologist, it unravels the mysteries and complexities of cancer treatment to the lay public. Its straightforward, down-to-earth style gives clear, sensible answers to questions that only a concerned physician rendering daily care to cancer patients can provide. Here is a book that gives reasons for coping and hoping with cancer. Its reading should be a requirement for all those concerned with cancer and its impact on living.

MORTON COLEMAN, M.D.
Director, Fund for Blood and Cancer Research
Associate Professor of Medicine and
Associate Director, Oncology Service
Cornell University Medical College

Preface

For a long time I have been aware of the urgent need for a readable, concise book to answer the questions frequently asked by cancer patients, their families, and the general public regarding the treatment of various types of cancer. What I have written here answers those questions and describes today's improved methods of cancer treatment, with emphasis on chemotherapy. The purpose of this book is to bring into sharp focus the great progress that has been made in the treatment of cancer and to describe the many areas where the battle against cancer is being won decisively. I hope to make people aware that the progress made in the treatment of one type of cancer leads to advances in the treatment of others, which ultimately will lead to a greater number of permanent cures.

My goal has been to present this vital information in a nontechnical, lucid form for the lay person as well as for health-care professionals. I have explained cancer and current advances in cancer treatment through case studies, drawings and photographs. With better understanding and up-to-date information, those touched by or concerned with cancer will be better equipped to cope with the disease in a rational manner.

Most books written on this subject are either too technical for the lay person or are filled mainly with anecdotal accounts that offer no really useful information to new cancer patients. In addition, the well-publicized controversies surrounding the treatment of cancer only add to the confusion of the patient and others concerned with cancer. What I am offering here is answers to the many concerns of cancer patients and their families—questions not always asked, and too often unanswered. This information is what patients not only need, but have a right to know.

This book also is intended to alleviate much of the desperation and hopelessness that most cancer patients experience during some stage of their illness because of lack of information. Accurate information will make it possible for patients to seek appropriate care early, which in turn will result in improved disease control. There is no question that cancer is still a major scourge; however, the significant recent achievements in its treatment make it possible for many patients to enjoy long-term remission and, in many instances, permanent cures. What I offer here are not exaggerated or false expectations but realistic understanding and hope.

VINCENT ANKU, M.D.
Southwest General Hospital
Middleburg Heights, Ohio

Acknowledgments

This book began as a small pamphlet that my wife, Yasmin, and I prepared for our patients. I must express my deepest appreciation to her and to our children, Kwame, Khama and Kofi, for their encouragement and support during the lengthy preparation of this work.

I am most grateful to Yasmin, Dr. Dorothy Martin and Mrs. Eloise Tressel for their help in making this book truly one for the lay person. I gratefully acknowledge the help of Doctors John Feldmann, Vishwa Sharan, James Hewlett and Joseph Wall, and of Mrs. Terry Mihelich, who all generously gave their time to read the manuscript and offer important suggestions. I deeply appreciate the editorial help of Dr. Ted Doering and the excellent foreword by Dr. Morton Coleman. I am greatly indebted to Mr. Willard Richmond for taking all the photographs, to Mr. Danny Carver for the excellent graphics and illustrations, and to the several secretaries whose skillful work made preparation of the manuscript much easier.

I will always treasure my association, nearly a decade so far, with my patients. To all of them I offer many thanks, because their courage has been the source for the optimism that is woven throughout this book. Since cancer treatment is always a team effort, special thanks go to all my colleagues, especially those at Metropolitan General Hospital and Cleveland Clinic, who have always been eager to offer their assistance and knowledge in helping care for my patients. I do appreciate the help of the dedicated nurses and the highly skilled radiologists and able referring physicians who have greatly supported my work, especially Doctors Martin Taliak, Charles Hoyt, Leopold Magpoc, Richard Pressler and Mohan Patel. Special thanks to Reverend and Mrs. Walter Trost and to Doctors Thomas Daniel, Daryush Haghighi, John Harris, John Hines, and Ali Shaikh and the late Dean Lawrence Hanlon for their help in my education and professional advancement. I owe a special debt to Southwest General Hospital and St. John and Westshore Hospital for their continuing support. Special thanks also to my publisher, and especially Sara Levant, for their enthusiasm and assistance.

Finally, I am indebted to Grinnell College and Cornell University for the full scholarships that enabled me to obtain an excellent education and to prepare for my career in medicine. I am particularly grateful to Dr. Martin Taliak and to my parents for their generosity and invaluable support over the years.

Contents

WHAT TO KNOW ABOUT

THE TREATMENT OF CANCER

CHAPTER ONE

Hope

You have just been told that you have cancer. Or that a loved one or a valued friend has cancer. Your initial shock, then panic and despair, are understandable. But I hope to be able to offer optimistic and realistic information to make it easier for you to deal with the physical as well as the emotional and social realities of the discovery.

This book will provide evidence from case histories that a cancer patient can indeed have realistic hopes for an extended, comfortable, useful life and even a cure. Progress is being made constantly in the battle against cancer and, as you will discover, some of the newer methods of treatment—even though they may not have made newspaper headlines—have had profound and positive effects on the lives of cancer patients. Specifically, these advances have taken place in radiation and, particularly, chemotherapy. I will discuss several types of cancer, including those that have proved to be treatable or curable—a category that includes some types of leukemia, lymph-node cancers (lymphomas), cancers of the reproductive organs (testicles and ovaries), and breast cancer.

Cancers That Are Especially Treatable

The rate of cure of certain types of leukemia in children now approaches 60 percent. The main reason for this encouraging percentage is the skillful use of various chemotherapeutic drugs in combination, a treatment method that has been in use only for about the past twenty years. Equally important has been the improvement in protecting patients from the undesirable and sometimes serious side effects of the medications. I know of many former leukemia patients who have finished school and now have families of their own, without any lingering effects of the disease.

Another milestone in the successful treatment of cancer is Hodgkin's disease. This cancer of the lymph nodes, which tends to attack patients in the prime of life, is now curable in 80 percent of all the patients who have it. This remarkable improvement is again due to the improved effectiveness of chemotherapy.

There have also been major advances in the treatment of cancer of the testicles since the late 1970s. This disease of young men used to result in a high death rate. Now, however, the rate of cure has dramatically jumped to 70 percent and over, even in advanced stages of the disease, and nearly 100 percent permanent, complete remission is possible in moderately advanced cases of testicular cancer treated with chemotherapy.

Effective use of chemotherapy has also improved the quality and rate of cure of breast cancer in recent years. Chemotherapy is now employed effectively in moderately advanced breast cancer that has spread to the lymph nodes. When all visibly involved lymph nodes are removed by surgery, and chemotherapy is administered with the goal of eradicating microscopic residual cancer cells, the chances of eventual relapse are greatly reduced.

Hope for the Future

If the current rate of progress in cancer treatment and research continues, ways to control the major killers, like cancer of the colon and the lung, will result in further sharp drops in deaths due to cancer. Because of the combination of surgery, radiation, and chemotherapy available today, the overall rate of cure for *all* cancers now is estimated to be 45 to 50 percent. *Cancer is now the most curable of all chronic diseases, and experts no longer regard cancer as the largely incurable disease it once was.* A reasonably early diagnosis and *correct* treatment from the onset could increase the rate of cure another 10 to 20 percent. Even those cancer patients who cannot be cured *can now live active, normal lives, with the disease under control for years,* assuming their cases are properly treated.

4

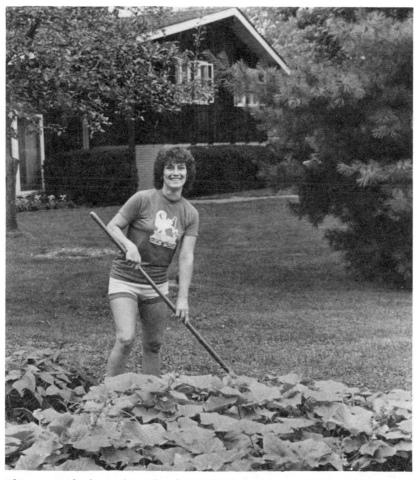

This woman had a moderately advanced cancer that was diagnosed in December, 1976 and was treated early and aggressively and has not returned, and she in all probability is cured. This woman's case is described on page 38.

Note: A professional photographer who was diagnosed in May 1980 and treated for bone cancer prepared all the photographs of the drawings and X rays used here.

Surgery and radiation, which are most successful in cases that have been detected early, are now being supplemented—with increasing success—by the use of chemotherapy. (*Chemotherapy* is exactly what its name suggests: treatment through the use of various chemicals.) Since chemotherapy is now playing a greater role than

Importance of Chemotherapy

5

ever in the treatment of cancer and will continue to be the central method of treatment of advanced cancer in the foreseeable future, the emphasis of this book is on chemotherapy: its usefulness and limitations. For anyone concerned with cancer, it is vital to understand the many aspects of chemotherapy as well as the use of various treatment techniques in combination. In addition to explaining chemotherapy in some detail, I will be describing the treatment of specific kinds of cancer and drawing on cases from my own experience and occasionally from experiences of my colleagues as illustrations.

But before going on to technical and specific information, I urge you to:

- Accept cancer as a chronic condition that can be treated;
- Maintain a positive attitude toward the very real possibility of successful treatment; and
- Read the following chapters carefully so that you can be fully informed not only about what is involved but also about what the patient can do for the success of the treatment.

Be aware, however, that this optimistic account of cancer treatment is not in any way intended to imply that science has conquered cancer or that cancer is close to being eliminated.

An important part of this book is the careful highlighting of significant new developments in cancer treatment. In many instances, the sense of inevitable doom and despair once associated with a diagnosis of cancer is not at all justified. If patients and their families and friends are fully informed about these new advances, they will seek *early* and *proper* help, which will improve their chances of survival and of normal lives.

CHAPTER TWO

Cancer: What It Is and How It Spreads

In order to understand cancer treatment, it is important to understand what cancer is. Cancer is *not* a single disease; there are, in fact, about 300 different types of cancer and many subdivisions within those types.

Cancer originates from a single or a few abnormally growing body cells. A cell is the smallest unit of the human body. Our bodies grow by division of individual cells. When a cell has reached its maximum size, it divides into two identical daughter cells—that is, two complete new cells (see illustration, following page). Cell division continues until the body stops growing. When the body reaches adult size, some distinct parts still retain the ability to keep dividing, particularly to replace the cells that wear out and die. The parts of the body that retain this ability include the hair, the skin, and the cells in the digestive system, blood, and damaged liver (liver cells may be damaged by hepatitis or excessive alcohol consumption).

Cell Division

Cancer cells are not foreign cells, but are part of our own bodies. A slow-growing cancer may stay for many years within the confines of, for example, the tissue of the prostate. In fact, in men over sixty,

Cancer Cells: Part of the Body

7

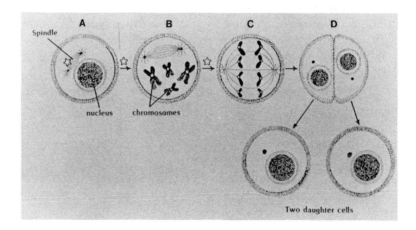

Stages of cell division. **A** shows the cell in the resting stage; material in the nucleus is semi-liquid. Cell division begins at **B,** with material in the nucleus condensed into pairs of strands called chromosomes. At **C,** the pairs of strands have separated into single strands, have attached themselves to the separated spindle and are moving toward opposite poles. At **D,** there are now two nuclei, each in a semi-liquid state, before the final division into two daughter cells.

Stars indicate stages where chemotherapy interferes with cell division.

perhaps 25 percent have small prostate cancers, but only a small percentage of those men will ever need treatment. Up to 30 percent of elderly males examined after death have "subclinical" prostate cancer (that is, cancer that never caused problems or resulted in medical treatment). Similarly, autopsies in Sweden revealed thyroid cancer in 9 percent of 500 patients forty to ninety years old, although the incidence in Sweden of thyroid cancer requiring treatment was only 5 per 100,000 (.005%) in women and 2 per 100,000 (.002%) in men. Many of us may have cancer cells but we do not have health problems because the body's natural defense (immunological) system is able to control their destructive tendencies.

Rapid Growth of Cancer Cells   A person is medically diagnosed as having cancer when that person's defense system is not functioning effectively. Only when the immunological system breaks down do the cancer cells acquire their unusual ability to proliferate much faster than other cells and start spreading. Normal cells do not grow at the same rapid pace as cancer cells. The rapid growth of cancer cells through unusually fast division is an exaggeration of normal bodily processes. During their abnormal growth, cancer cells crowd out normal cells and, as they increase in size, they press on normal tissues or nerves, which can cause pain.

Although cancer cells tend to grow fast, the speed at which they grow varies from tumor to tumor. (The words *tumor* and *cancer* will be used in this book interchangeably.) Some grow so fast that the cancer can double in size every twenty-four hours (as, for example, in Burkitt's lymphoma). Another example is small-cell cancer of the lung, which can double in size every three weeks.

On the other hand, some tumors can take as long as 100 to 200 days to double in size. Some types of breast cancer can take over eight years from the time the cells become cancerous to the time they become detectable.

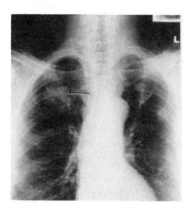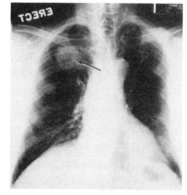

A slow-growing lung cancer. Arrows point to a tumor (white area) shown on X rays taken in November, 1980 and October, 1983. (The large white area in the center and toward the right is the heart.)

Cancer has several major distinguishing features. First are the abnormal cells that are growing very fast and eventually develop into a detectable mass. A second major characteristic is the disorder of the cells' growth; as a rule, a cancer does not have well-defined boundaries. Third, these cells have the unusual ability to travel from their place of origin to other parts of the body, where they may rest until they start growing again under the "right" conditions. Tumors that are growing relatively slowly tend to keep growing but have very little tendency to travel to other places until they reach an advanced

Special Traits of Cancer

stage. The unique feature of cancer that enables it to travel and grow in distant parts of the body is called *metastasis*. This is the special characteristic that distinguishes a *malignant*—cancerous—tumor from a *benign*—noncancerous—one (see photographs, page 13).

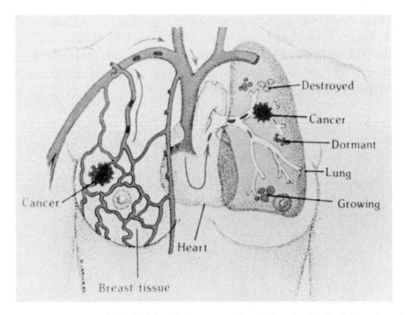

How cancers spread via the blood. Cancer cells originating in the breast break off from the parent tumor and travel to the heart. From there they might travel to other organs, where they may be destroyed by the body's defense mechanism, or may start growing, or stay dormant for months or years.

How Metastasis Takes Place   One way that tumors metastasize is via the blood vessels. Cancer cells are carried in the blood to other parts of the body such as the liver, lungs, or bones. The other important means of spreading is by the lymph system, which consists of the lymph channel and the lymph nodes. The lymph channel is made up of small spaces in the body tissues where fluid that has leaked out of the blood vessels is collected and eventually taken back into circulation. Foreign or abnormal particles such as cancer cells can be picked up in the lymph channel and taken to the lymph nodes, which are scattered at strategic locations all over the body (in the neck, armpits, chest, abdomen, and groin, for example). The main function of the lymph nodes is to destroy foreign or abnormal bodies such as bacteria or cancerous

10

cells. Different parts of the body have their own lymph channels and nodes. The lymph from the breast tends to drain its fluid first into the lymph nodes under the arm or near the center of the rib cage (the sternum) or below and above the collar bone (the clavicle). This is why the lymph nodes under the arm or around the rib cage or collar bone become involved early when breast cancer is spreading. The drawing on page 12 shows a tumor inside the lymph channels in the breast tissue. From the breast the cancer cells migrate into the lymph channel and eventually may enter the lymph node, where they may be destroyed or may start to grow.

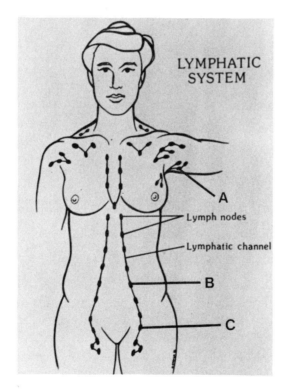

The lymph system.

A woman with a breast tumor may therefore have cancer that has spread to the lymph glands or nodes under the arm, or to the liver, bones, or other parts of the body. This does not mean that the cancerous breast tumor has grown and spread like an amoeba moving

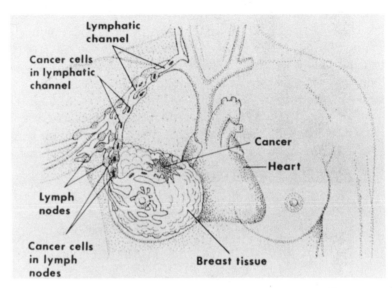

Lymph drainage of the breast, showing another way cancer cells can travel.

directly from the breast to the armpit, involving all the tissues between the two. Rather, it means that breast-cancer cells are able to break away from the parent cancer, invade the blood or lymph channels, and be carried to distant parts of the body. The lymph nodes that act as sieves may or may not allow the cancer cells to pass through. If the cells become lodged in the lymph nodes and conditions are favorable to the cells, they will begin to grow and lymph-node involvement, or *lymph-node metastasis*, has taken place. Similarly, if the cell is able to pass through the lymph nodes, it may or may not find another favorable place to grow in. Many cancer cells are killed in transit by our own defense mechanisms before having the opportunity to become lodged in other parts of the body.

How Tumor Size Affects Metastasis

The size of a tumor usually influences its chances of metastasizing; the larger the tumor, the more likely it is to spread. This is why it is critically important to detect and deal with a tumor early.

Why Treatment Varies

It is also important to be aware that the problems caused by cancer depend upon the type, the location, and the pattern of

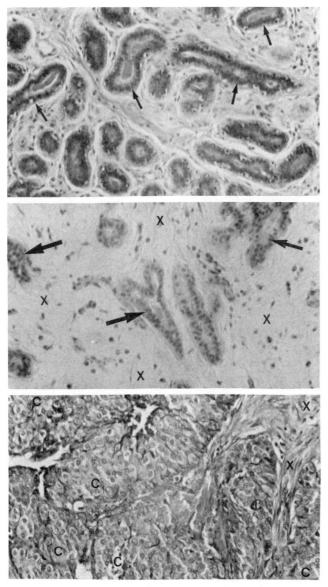

Normal, benign and cancerous breast tissue. *Top:* normal breast tissue, with two well-defined components, the milk glands (arrows) and connective tissue. *Center:* benign breast tumor, where the connective tissue (*X*) has spread and the number of milk glands is reduced. *Bottom:* cancerous breast tissue, with the milk glands and connective tissue combined into a large mass of cancerous cells (*C*) and no longer separately identifiable.

spreading. Even cancers in the same location (for example, any of the many types of lung cancer) can grow and spread at different rates. Consequently, no two patients have exactly the same condition. Therefore, the type of treatment appropriate for one patient may not necessarily benefit another who appears to have a similar situation. Tumors that are growing relatively slowly and would have a tendency to spread late may require only surgery for a cure, if treated early. On

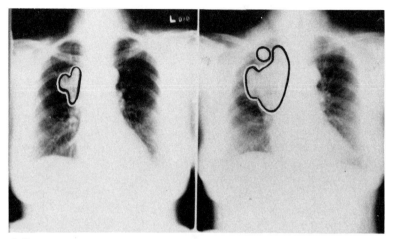

A fast-growing cancer. X rays were taken in December, 1979 and in January, 1980.

the other hand, tumors that have a tendency to grow very rapidly and spread early cannot be cured by surgery or radiation alone. Chemotherapy is particularly useful in treating the second, rapidly-growing type of tumor because chemical agents can travel to all parts of the body through the blood stream and lymph channels. This results in generalized treatment rather than the localized approach that surgery and radiation offer.

There is a second reason why chemotherapy is effective on a fast-growing tumor: chemotherapy destroys a large percentage of dividing cancer cells and makes them unable to reproduce daughter cells. The only way cancer cells, which are relatively weak, can do their damage is by sheer volume. Because of their feeble nature, cancer cells have relatively little ability to regenerate when they are attacked by radiation or chemicals. Normal cells, on the other hand, have a greater ability to recuperate and recover from the effects of

14

chemotherapy. This is why chemotherapy is so much more devastating to cancer cells and has a lasting effect on them. Obviously, the more researchers can learn about the differences between normal cells and cancer cells, the greater will be our ability to use chemotherapy effectively to attack and overcome the cancer cells.

CHAPTER THREE

Choosing A Specialist

The majority of cancer patients in the United States and Canada receive good to excellent medical care. But, in spite of easy access to competent treatment, a significant percentage of cancer patients are simply not receiving adequate care. This chapter will help the concerned person select the best physician for his or her particular situation. It is absolutely necessary to find the right doctor because the quality of care and the end result depend very much on the competence of the physicians involved.

Getting
the Right Help Early

The major reason why many curable cancers become uncontrollable is delay in diagnosis. Also, in some instances, treatment may be inadequate or improper after diagnosis. It is, clearly, very important to *seek proper help immediately when a cancer has been discovered.* In the majority of cases where the cancer has spread beyond the organ of origin, surgery alone cannot produce a cure. Patients in this situation require highly specialized and comprehensive care. It is at the time of diagnosis that the patient should seek *expert* advice if none is provided or arranged by the attending physician. The successful treatment of cancer is highly complicated and delicate, requiring very careful planning and thorough knowledge of the many aspects of the treatment of specific cancers. Several important factors must be taken into account in determining the proper treatment and medications to be used for any given person. Such factors would include the age, sex and overall physical state of the patient as well as the behavior of the particular tumor. It is no exaggeration to say that the treatment of certain cancers is more complicated than open-heart surgery. Clearly, for the best results it is extremely important for patients to go directly to physicians who are thoroughly experienced in cancer treatment.

Even though cancer is a very important public-health problem, the disease did not receive proper attention in any part of the world until the 1970s. Since then, however, there has been a tremendous commitment to fighting cancer. The advances in cancer treatment in recent years have been due to improved surgical techniques as well as better radiation treatment and the availability of more effective cancer-fighting medications. However, the single most important recent advance has been the training of thousands of experts to care for cancer patients, thanks to dedicated medical educators and pioneers who recognized the urgent need to provide such expertise to their own communities. This trend has resulted in the availability of many dedicated and specially trained physicians, nurses, social-service personnel and volunteers who work very hard to make life worthwhile for the cancer patient.

The Biggest Step Forward — Cancer Specialists

It is noteworthy that one of the foremost pioneers in cancer treatment, Dr. James Ewing, saw the need for training cancer specialists as early as the late 1920s. He realized that the average physician did not recognize the uniqueness of cancer as a lethal disease. Untreated, cancer invariably causes death. But this outcome, as Ewing recognized, can be dramatically turned around by early diagnosis and proper, timely action to a degree that applies to no other major cause of death. He concluded that cancer treatment had arrived at a point where it required specific training: the treatment of cancer should be done by specialists.

Yet it was not until the early 1970s that cancer-specialist training programs were started and *oncology*—the study of cancer—became a word familiar to the layman. Programs for training adult medical

Cancer Specialists' Training

cancer specialists were started first, followed by programs for pediatric cancer specialists. Both the adult and the pediatric cancer-specialist programs require five to six years of additional training after medical school. After this training, doctors take a national examination, the American Boards in Medical/Pediatric Oncology. After passing this rigorous exam, they become Board Certified Oncologists. There are a few good cancer specialists who are not Board certified. However, for the patient or family searching for a specialist, Board certification of an M.D. as an oncologist is a good yardstick for measuring the level of expertise.

Physicians Specializing in Cancer

There are now specialists in various fields of cancer treatment: the adult medical oncologist, pediatric oncologist, radiation oncologist, gynecological oncologist, and surgical oncologist. The following is a brief description of each.

The Adult Medical Oncologist

The most appropriate physician to take care of an adult with cancer is the *adult medical oncologist*. These physicians specialize in overseeing all the treatment of an adult who has cancer—even though they themselves may not be the specialists who give all the treatment. They are not only qualified to determine the best type of treatment for a particular cancer, but they are also experienced in the complications of cancer that would not be apparent to a doctor who is not an oncologist. I should emphasize that medical oncologists are not surgeons; they do not operate. They are certified in internal medicine and treat other adult illnesses such as diabetes, high blood pressure, anemia and so on, as well as cancer. The adult medical oncologist is also familiar with the various resources—social and financial—that are available to cancer patients. In the hands of a properly trained oncologist, the patient is most likely to receive the most up-to-date care both in major medical centers and in local community hospitals, as well as profiting from any unique resources that are available.

The Pediatric Oncologist

The *pediatric oncologist* specializes in the diseases of children and, in addition, in the care of cancers that occur in children. In both the U.S. and Canada there are so far only a few pediatric oncologists, and they tend to work at university hospitals or major medical centers. However, recent progress in the treatment of childhood cancers has been phenomenal, and many childhood cancers are now completely curable. It is, therefore, essential to take a child to a well-qualified pediatric oncologist to insure getting the best possible chance for a cure. If you are a parent who finds there are no such specialists in your area, you can start with an adult medical oncologist, who should then work in consultation, via the telephone, with a pediatric oncologist. This type of cooperation between two oncologists in different locations has been successful. However, difficult pediatric cases should be treated only by those most qualified to provide the best possible care, and you may have to travel to wherever that care is. In such situations, hospitals can sometimes help out regarding housing.

Radiation oncologists, who have extensive training in treating cancer with radiation, work closely with other oncologists. The complications of radiation therapy have been greatly reduced since the mid-'70s because of the refinement of new equipment and a strong emphasis on proper training. I have seen only two serious skin burns from radiation during the last ten years, even though I have referred large numbers of patients for such treatment. And both of the burns healed well.

The Radiation Oncologist

Gynecological oncologists are gynecological surgeons who specialize in the total care of women who have cancer of the ovary, uterus, cervix or related areas. These physicians take three to four years' training after medical school in addition to two more years' training in the treatment of cancers in women. They are able to do surgery as well as give chemotherapy. In addition, they can give some forms of internal radiation, but not external radiation. There are only a few gynecological oncologists in the U.S. Some cancers of the female reproductive system can be handled perfectly well by an adult medical oncologist, but unusual and difficult cases should be referred to a gynecological oncologist.

The Gynecological Oncologist

The *surgical oncologist* is a surgeon skilled in performing cancer surgery in addition to having expertise in giving chemotherapy after surgery. Again, there are only a few of these specialists and they are usually at very large institutions. Skilled though they are, surgical oncologists, even at the most prestigious hospitals, invariably refer their patients to adult medical oncologists after surgery because of the numerous problems associated with cancer and the need for treatment that surgeons would not be well equipped to handle. Even in a few cases where the surgeon decides to remain in charge of all aspects of treatment (including administering chemotherapy), this is often done with the cooperation of a medical oncologist.

Patients should be warned that there is a recent and dangerous trend in community clinics and hospitals where some physicians have declared themselves to be oncologists practically overnight and have decided to provide total care for patients after diagnosis or surgery. The majority of these physicians have not had much training in treating cancer. Some of them may have worked in a cancer ward for three or four months during their surgical training and hence feel that they can now qualify as cancer specialists. A situation may arise when there is no cancer specialist available in a particular area to provide care for cancer patients, and an internist or general surgeon may reluctantly assume the job and do the best work possible. However, physicians in this situation are quite willing to transfer patients to an oncologist as soon as one becomes available. The real problem is physicians who are totally untrained but refuse to refer the patients for expert care that is readily available. Though it is only a small number of physicians who engage in such practices, the havoc they cause in terms of physical and economic suffering is enormous. These doctors as a group are usually not busy and are trying to "branch out" to make extra income at the expense of the cancer patients.

I can recall a case that underscores the importance of selecting a qualified oncologist—a case where a seemingly hopeless situation was completely reversed and resulted in several years of normal and comfortable life.

This case illustrates what can be accomplished when the proper steps are taken immediately. The patient, the family doctor, and the attending surgeon each acted promptly; in addition, the surgeon sought help right away by referring the patient to a medical oncologist. The medical oncologist in turn got appropriate help to provide the best possible care for the patient.

A sixty-four-year-old man was hospitalized in April, 1980 for abdominal pain and diarrhea that had lasted for two weeks. X rays showed that he had a huge tumor of the lower colon. During exploratory surgery, it was found that the tumor had made holes in the colon at several points and had formed numerous channels into the small intestines, with extensive local metastasis and lymph-node involvement. The surgeon did an excellent job of removing the bulk of the cancer and immediately referred the patient to the oncologist, who referred him to a radiation oncologist to treat the remaining tumor in the pelvis and lower abdomen. The patient tolerated the radiation very well without any side effects.

Dramatic Response to New Drugs

After the radiation the oncologist started the patient on chemotherapy. This time the patient did well for only about five months; then he started showing signs of a small-bowel obstruction that grew very quickly and caused constant diarrhea, nausea and vomiting. The patient's condition began to deteriorate rapidly. The following December, when the patient was being readmitted, the hospital staff could easily see the anguish and pain in the eyes of his wife because she assumed that her husband would not leave the hospital alive. Examination showed the patient had small-bowel obstructions at numerous sites, making surgery or additonal radiation out of the question. The oncologist placed him on very aggressive chemotherapy while carefully monitoring the complications. The patient responded dramatically to the new combination of chemotherapeutic drugs and ever since then has enjoyed significant remission and has led a full, active life. The photograph on the following page was taken more than four years after his initial diagnosis.

Most nonspecialists treating this patient would have started the first stage of chemotherapy after surgery and continued it every week. When it was no longer effective (in this case about eight months after surgery), they might have told the patient and the family, "We have done everything possible and nothing further can be done." The patient would have died six to eight months after radiation therapy.

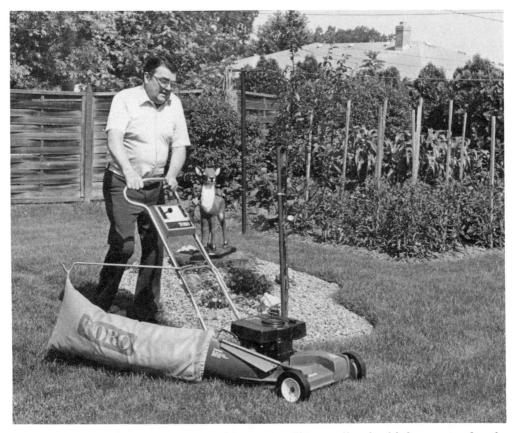

Colon cancer patient. This man is still in excellent health four years after the initial diagnosis of his disease. Among his interests is his thriving vegetable garden, only partially shown here.

Specialized treatment in this case accomplished two goals: Radiation prevented an early return of the cancer in the pelvic region, which would have caused bladder damage and bleeding during urination. Eventually there would have been kidney blockage and destruction. Second, and most important, the compression and pinching of pelvic nerves, which would have caused considerable pain, were also prevented. The oncologist, when the first chemotherapy treatment failed, was able to administer more potent medications in a new combination and successfully manage the serious complications. This kind of knowledge is far beyond that of most nonspecialists who attempt to treat cancer of the colon. Although there is no cure for advanced colon cancer at the present time, aggressive and proper treatment, such as took place in this case, can offer extra months—or years—of activity.

A valuable point I should make here is that when a patient has a qualified oncologist, the patient is really getting a team; as in this case, the physician will call in whatever other specialists are needed to help, and the skill and knowledge are multiplied several times.

Teamwork in Treatment

It must be stressed that successful results in the treatment of cancer require a great deal of expertise and cannot be accomplished by physicians who dabble in cancer care and have not received proper and adequate training. It is ironic that there is so much fuss about the cancer quackery performed by people providing unproven drugs for cancer treatment when greater quackery is committed by a few untrained physicians who are using proven drugs improperly. Very little is being done or can be done to protect patients who are the victims in this second situation. It is left to an informed public to demand the right to be treated by competent specialists.

CHAPTER FOUR

Major Types
of Cancer Treatment

The major types of cancer treatment are surgery, radiation and chemotherapy, and they can be used separately or in various combinations. This chapter will describe each method and its usefulness.

Surgery

Surgery is the oldest and still the number-one method of treating cancer. Until recently it was the only method for a sure cure because it involved removing all cancerous cells early before they had a chance to spread. Specifically, surgery is used for diagnosis and treatment in three ways:

- *Biopsy*—the removal of a piece or all of the tumor for examination and diagnosis.
- *Staging*—the examination of other tissues, following a biopsy, so the physician can determine the full extent and spread of the tumor. For example, the spleen may be removed in a case of Hodgkin's disease in order to determine whether the cancer was in an early or advanced stage and thus whether radiation and/or chemotherapy should be used.

24

- *Treatment*—surgery performed either to cure the disease or to ease it (palliative surgery), that is, to prevent or eliminate some effects of the tumor. For example, *curative surgery* is done when cancer is still confined to the wall of the colon and has not spread, but *palliative surgery* is performed for colon cancer even if the tumor has spread in order to prevent the patient from later developing a bowel obstruction.

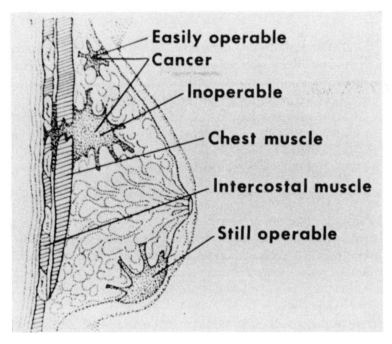

Operable and inoperable tumors. In some cases an initially inoperable tumor can be shrunk by radiation or chemotherapy and then surgically removed.

As a general rule, with only a few exceptions such as colon cancer, surgery is not advisable when the tumor has already spread. But occasionally, even though there is widespread metastasis, a surgeon may remove the primary cancer in order to relieve symptoms. Examples would be breast removal (mastectomy) or removal of a cancerous kidney that is bleeding excessively. A patient with cancer that has spread to several areas of the body is not a candidate for surgery because it is impossible to remove all the tumors from

25

various areas. Besides, there may be locations where the cells are present but not yet visible, where they will surely start growing after surgery. There is no point in removing the primary tumor, since the patient's problems may be due more to the effects of metastasis than to the tumor itself. Surgical treatment of cancer, therefore, is most suitable in situations where the cancer is growing slowly and would metastasize late. When surgery is performed in such cases, before the tumor spreads, the chances of cure are excellent.

Importance of Early Detection
The advantages of early detection are obvious. Solitary tumors do not cause problems except for local pressure; if such tumors are removed at this point, symptoms will be eliminated and there will be good chance of a cure. In 85 percent of the cases of breast cancer that has not spread, surgery alone has been all that was needed to effect a cure. I know of a patient who had cancer of the colon and severe anemia. Detection was early (before there was any spread), so the patient required only surgery. This woman now, nearly eight years later, has no evidence of metastasis and can be considered cured.

Surgery Combined with Other Treatment
Surgery when combined with radiation and/chemotherapy is useful in treating certain cancers such as those of the head and neck, and of the ovaries. Even though many such tumors are initially inoperable, they can be reduced in size by radiation or chemotherapy and thus made operable.

Most well-trained general surgeons should be able to perform cancer surgery. However, many tumors — such as those of the throat, lung, brain and, in rare cases, the liver — require special training for proper surgical treatment. The most important point here is what is done *after* surgery. A patient may not require any further treatment, but far more often patients who should have radiation or chemotherapy to achieve a complete cure or long-term remission are told, "We've gotten it all." The result is that no further treatment is given and the tumor returns in a few months or years. I strongly recommend that a patient consult an oncologist at the time of diagnosis rather than wait until later in the course of treatment.

An experienced surgeon doing a routine operation should not have unusual problems. All problems from surgery, whether cancer is involved or not, depend on the location of the tumor and the skill of the surgeon. An "easy" operation is less likely to develop complications than a more complex one.

Radiation is the process in which cancer cells are damaged or destroyed through bombardment with minute high-energy particles that are smaller than atoms. Radiation therapy is playing an increasingly useful role in the treatment of cancer—in fact, about half of the cancer patients who have been treated have received radiation therapy at some stage. Radiation has limitations; like surgery, it is useful for local treatment but is less effective for tumors that have spread.

When the energy of radiation passes through a particular cell, it can cause disorganization of the atomic particles within the cell that are involved in cell division. In particular, it affects the delicate structures within the DNA particles—the chains that determine which characteristics of a cell will be inherited. Hence, like chemotherapy, radiation attacks cancer cells by disrupting the process of cell division. Since cancer cells are dividing at a faster rate than normal cells, the cancer cells are more vulnerable to radiation than normal cells. Also, normal cells have a greater ability to repair the damage done by radiation than do cancer cells. A particular cancer is said to be especially *radiosensitive* if only a small dose of radiation is required to kill it. In this case little damage is done to the normal cells. On the other hand, cancer cells that are *radioresistant* require tremendous amounts of radiation to kill them, which means that there is a small margin of safety for normal cells.

Medical scientists do not know why certain types of cells are more sensitive than others to radiation. They know very well, however, what dose of radiation is needed for temporary control of symptoms or for permanent control of various cancerous tissues. They also know quite precisely how much radiation various vital organs can safely receive.

The dose of radiation used on body tissues is measured in units called *rads*. Some tumors of the testicle that are very radiosensitive (for example, seminomas) require only about 3,000 rads in order for

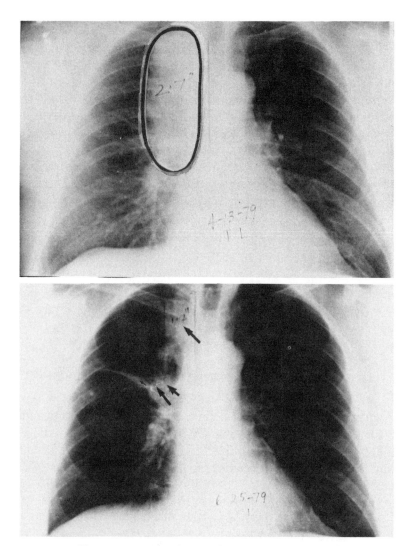

Response of lung cancer to radiation therapy. Top X ray, taken in April 1979, shows a tumor nearly three inches in diameter covering 25 percent of the upper chest. X ray below was taken in June, 1979, after radiation. Of the original tumor, only scar tissue (arrows) remains.

the disease to be eradicated, whereas tumors of the muscles, which are classified as radioresistant, may require up to 8,000 rads. Between these two extremes, different cancers exhibit various degrees of radiosensitivity.

28

The results of radiation can be quite dramatic. The X rays in the illustration show a massive lung cancer (adenocarcinoma) approximately 3 by 5 inches in size in the upper right chest. The patient received a carefully planned high dose of radiation (6,000 rads) that completely destroyed the tumor. Except for slight fatigue, he experienced no side effects from the radiation and continued to work full time during the treatment. More important, the tumor in the chest was destroyed and the patient has experienced no more chest problems.

The goal of radiation therapy, when used early for diseases that are very radiosensitive, is to achieve permanent cures or at least give significant relief from the symptoms. Permanent cures can be achieved with early tumors of the head and neck as well as certain tumors of the testicle. In the first stage of Hodgkin's disease, a cure can be expected in 90 percent of the cases with radiation therapy alone.

In addition to treating the cancer directly, radiation also plays a major role in relieving unpleasant symptoms. It is particularly useful in relieving pressure, obstruction, and pain (especially in the spinal cord or breathing tubes). In cases of pressure on the spinal cord, timely radiation, by destroying the tumor, can prevent paralysis of the legs.

Improvements in Radiation Treatment

Since the early '70s, radiation treatment has improved considerably for several reasons. First, there has been a significant improvement in the quality of the equipment. The old X-ray equipment produced low-energy radiation measured in thousand-volt units called *kilovolts* or *orthovolts*. Orthovoltage equipment, which had many faults, gave radiation therapy a bad name. The equipment did not have great ability to go through tissue nor could it be aimed very accurately at the tumor. There was, therefore, considerable random scattering of radiation energy into the skin and tissue surrounding the tumor, which resulted in severe skin burns and injury to normal cells. The newer equipment produces energy levels so high that they are measured in millions of volts—*megavolts* or *supervolts*. Megavoltage radiation is better able to penetrate tissue so that the skin is now spared. When the chemical element cobalt, with its exceptionally intense gamma-ray activity, was discovered, it was used to further reduce many of the problems previously resulting from orthovoltage radiation.

Today's newer equipment includes linear accelerators, which provide very high radiation energy and can be beamed at the tumor with great accuracy. And machines that beam electrons are even more versatile. These can be directed more precisely at certain depths, and therefore are invaluable for radiating the skin and difficult areas such as the eyelid, where damage to the eye itself must be avoided. This type of radiation allows the doctor to radiate the same area several times at various intervals without damage to important internal organs. This is particularly useful for patients who have breast cancer with skin involvement and have had previous radiation therapy to the chest. Radiation can be performed in such a way that the bones and lungs can be spared from further exposure to radiation.

Radiation Given Early Another reason for the improved benefits of radiation therapy is that patients now receive it much earlier, when they can tolerate radiation better. In the past, radiation was applied as a last resort. Now radiation is used as an integral part of treatment aimed at cure or long-term remission.

Finally, rigorous training is now required of radiation oncologists. The steady improvement in equipment, early use of radiation, and special training of doctors have led to a significant reduction in complications and unpleasant side effects from radiation. Radiation can still result in complications or unpleasant side effects—depending on the location and dose of the radiation—but these are experienced today only by a small percentage of patients.

How Radiation When a patient is advised to have radiation, a radiation
Therapy is Given oncologist studies the case carefully and decides whether radiation will be beneficial. Assuming it will be, the doctor will discuss with the patient the type of radiation, duration, frequency and complications of the particular treatment.

After the consultation, the area of the patient's body to be included in the field of radiation will be clearly marked with indelible ink. The ink should not be washed off until the treatment has ended. During the actual radiation, the vital areas around the tumor may be protected with lead shields to prevent radiation injury.

A small dose of radiation (about 200 to 300 rads) is given each time the patient comes in for treatment. It may take only one to two minutes to deliver each dose. Radiation treatment is often given daily except on weekends and may require ten to twenty-five days, depending on the type of tumor, its location, and the goal of the treatment (whether it's curative or palliative). There is no pain or discomfort during the radiation, and the sensation is no different from having a chest X ray.

Some patients experience no side effects whatsoever. Others do, depending on the dose of radiation and the part of the body that receives it. There may be some general reactions such as fatigue, lack of energy and loss of appetite. Nausea may be experienced if radiation is given to the chest or abdomen. Low blood counts (a decrease in the number of blood cells) can occur if large parts of the body are included, especially areas where the blood is formed as, for example, the pelvic bone. A temporary break in the treatment schedule may be required for the patient who needs to recuperate from some of these side effects.

Side Effects of Radiation

The most common reaction to radiation is changes in the skin, which can range from mild redness to irritation or burns. Very severe skin reactions and radiation burns are rare today because of the quality of the new equipment, and most skin reactions can be easily treated with soothing lotions or baby powder. Itching and flaking, which are frequent reactions, can be treated with cornstarch or mild cortisone creams.

Temporary hair loss is the rule when the head is involved in radiation. However, if a tumor of the scalp requires heavy radiation to the skin, the hair loss that occurs may, in some cases, be permanent. A sore or dry mouth or throat could occur in varying degrees if the mouth or throat is included in the radiation field.

Tumors swell a bit following the first few radiation treatments. Cancers located in the brain, the spinal cord or in very small spaces in the body have little room for expansion. Therefore, symptoms of the disease could become worse after radiation of such tumors. This problem is temporary and may be avoided by moderately high doses of cortisone to help prevent initial swelling (edema) of the tumor.

High doses of radiation to the chest can cause inflammation of the heart lining (pericarditis) and result in chest pain, a problem that is usually short-lived. Radiation pneumonia occurs in a very small percentage of patients who receive high doses of radiation to the lung. This is accompanied by fever, coughing, fatigue, and profuse sweating. Radiation pneumonia may respond to brief treatment with cortisone, since this side effect is a form of inflammation.

Shielding During Radiation Treatment
During abdominal radiation, the vital organs in the abdomen such as the liver, kidney and small bowel, which cannot tolerate high doses of radiation, are protected or shielded. In younger women the ovaries are protected to prevent sterility. Often nausea and vomiting and, sometimes, diarrhea are experienced by patients undergoing abdominal radiation. A small percentage of patients who receive large doses end up with damage to the bowels called radiation colitis. However, by far the majority of patients who do develop diarrhea do not have it for long and may not require any treatment for it.

Why Radiation May Be Ineffective
Radiation may not always work on cancer cells because the cells can become radioresistant. There are two reasons why this can happen. First, conventional types of radiation such as X rays and gamma rays work best on cancer cells that are in areas of high oxygen. These cells, reasonably enough, are called *highly oxygenated cells* while those in low-oxygen areas are *hypoxic cells.* The central portion of most tumors has many hypoxic cells. Conventional radiation therapy can be almost completely ineffective in destroying the central portion of very large tumors.

The second major reason for resistance is that human cells have a tendency to repair themselves when exposed to radiation. Cancer cells, as I have already pointed out, as a whole have less capacity to recover from radiation damage than do normal cells. However, some cancer cells develop ways of recovering before the next dose of radiation, thus completely escaping any permanent damage. Since the central—hypoxic—portion of the tumor is less likely to receive adequate radiation anyway, the cancer cells in that area can more easily recover from the effect of radiation. This phenomenon again emphasizes the need for early detection and diagnosis: The smaller the cancer, the more easily it can be treated by any means, including radiation.

There are new developments which, though still in their infancy, can get around these two causes of radioresistance. One of these new developments, the *neutron beam*, can attack cancer cells that are well oxygenated as well as poorly oxygenated. The neutron beam also reduces the ability of cancer cells to repair radiation damage. In some studies of patients with head and neck tumors, nearly 80 percent of the tumors disappeared with fast-neutron-beam radiation, compared to 20 percent in conventional X-ray therapy.

The results are even more encouraging if conventional radiation is *combined* with fast-neutron radiation. Preliminary studies show that in addition to resulting in a better response, combination radiation also results in fewer complications. At this time, however, neutron treatment is still in an experimental stage and is available only in a very few cities in the world.

Counteracting Radioresistance

Chemotherapy—the treatment of cancer by various chemicals—is discussed in detail in the next chapter, so the discussion here is intended simply as an introduction to the subject.

Because cancer usually has spread by the time of the initial diagnosis, cure by surgery or radiation alone is probably not possible. Thus the need for chemotherapeutic drugs, which can travel via the blood stream and lymph channels and are able to pursue and destroy the cancer cells that have metastasized.

Chemotherapy

Chemotherapy kills cancer cells by depriving them of substances that they need for growth and cell division.

In order to divide, every cell produces a certain amount of DNA, which carries the basic material that determines what will be inherited. DNAs, which are acid chemical substances (D-nucleic acid), are located in the nucleus of the cell and are the fundamental constituents of chromosomes, which carry the genes. Under a special microscope, DNAs look like long beads threaded together to form the tapelike chromosomes. The DNAs contain all the information a cell needs to carry on all its vital functions. If a cell develops defective or insufficent DNAs, then its ability to function, as well as its ability to divide, is severely impaired. During cell division each DNA produces a replica of itself—double the amount of original DNA. Only at this

How Chemotherapy Works

point can the cell divide in two, with each daughter cell receiving an identical copy of the parent's DNA. If a cell is unable to produce the proper type or amount of DNA required by each daugher cell, the parent cell will die (see illustration).

The goal of chemotherapy, then, is to make it impossible for cancer cells to produce daughter cells. Chemotherapeutic drugs do this by:

- Interfering with the production of DNA at various stages in cell division, or
- Binding the DNA so tightly that it cannot divide to make a copy for each of the two daughter cells, or
- Depriving the cancer cells of certain amino acids that are essential for the nutrition and growth of cancer cells but are not needed by normal cells.

When chemotherapy is successful and stops the cancer cells from dividing, these cells begin to fall apart; the tumor stops growing and begins to shrink.

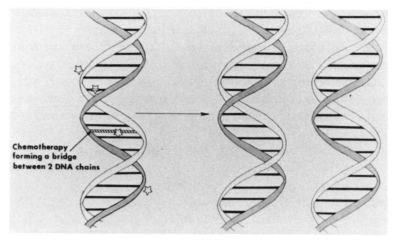

Chemotherapy forming a bridge between 2 DNA chains

How chemotherapy blocks cell division. Cancers grow by cell division; before any cell can divide, it must increase the amount of DNA it contains so that each daughter cell will carry the same hereditary information the parent carried. This drawing shows the basic structure of DNA: two threads twisted together like two strands of yarn and joined by units like the rungs of a ladder. Normally, the parent would produce the two daughter cells shown at right.

Chemotherapy interferes with the production of new DNA material (starred) that is needed for daughter cells. Chemotherapy can also form an un-breakable rung between the two strands of DNA (arrow), thus preventing formation of daughter DNAs and ultimately preventing cell division.

Chemotherapy is most successful if used when cancer cells are most vulnerable. Cancer cells do not all divide at the same time or rate, and some of them rest after division. Recently it has been learned that by combining various chemotherapeutic drugs and using them simultaneously, cancer cells can be attacked at various stages of division. Combination chemotherapy produces a more completely devastating effect on the cancer cells than single medications used separately. The number of cancer cells that can be killed by a combination of different chemotherapeutic drugs is high, and in many cases can lead to a more rapid shrinkage of the tumor.

Combination Chemotherapy

Combination chemotherapy is extremely useful for another important reason—the complexity and variety of cancer. Two patients may seem to have an identical type of cancer, but one may respond very well to treatment while the other may not. The reason lies partly in the variability of the cancer cells. There may be two or more varieties of cancer cells within the same tumor. One population may be very sensitive to certain chemicals while the other group of cells may be sensitive to entirely different chemicals. By using a combination of drugs, all of which may have proven to be effective against a particular tumor, the physician has a better chance of eliminating the different populations of cancerous cells.

It would be extremely helpful to know in advance precisely which chemicals will be effective for a particular patient so that those chemicals alone could be used. In research now under way, specimens of cancerous cells are cultured outside the body and tested against various chemotherapeutic drugs. Perfection of this testing technique will be a boon to cancer treatment, because physicians can then use specific medications that they know will be effective for individual patients. This will greatly improve results as well as reduce side effects.

Sometimes the goal of chemotherapy is to block sex hormones.

Anti-Estrogen Treatment

Certain human sex hormones stimulate the growth of many types of cancer. Research conclusively shows that ovarian hormones encourage the development of some breast tumors, both benign and malignant. These hormones—*estrogens*—cause growth because of their effect on the genes in a cell's nucleus. The estrogens bind onto a protein called *estrogen-receptor* in the cells. This results in a new estrogen, *estrogen-receptor complex*, which migrates into the cell nucleus, where it influences the cell growth and function. About 60 to 80 percent of human breast cancers have estrogen-receptor proteins. Anything that blocks the interaction between the estrogen and the estrogen-receptor protein can diminish the growth-stimulating effect of the estrogens. *Anti-estrogens* are now available that bind selectively to estrogen-receptors and block the formation of estrogen-receptor complexes. The higher the level of estrogen-receptor proteins, the better the anti-estrogen effect. A laboratory-produced anti-estrogen with the trade name Nolvadex (chemically known as tamoxifen) is very effective for treatment of breast cancer.

CHAPTER FIVE

How Chemotherapy Is Given

The treatment of cancer, whether with surgery, radiation or chemotherapy, is like going to war. The oncologist, like the military commander, has a better chance of winning the battle if he sends 10,000 troops against 5,000 enemies. This chapter will describe the battle that makes use of chemotherapy: the timing and methods of treatment.

Usually chemotherapy is started two to three weeks after surgery, which allows sufficient time for the patient to heal and regain strength. Chemotherapy too soon after surgery is not advisable because chemotherapy can slow down the healing, since chemotherapy affects dividing cells, which are involved in the healing process. Sometimes surgical complications such as infections can be another reason for not starting chemotherapy too soon. In addition to waiting for the surgery to heal, it is also important to build up the patient's strength through good nutrition before the additional stress of chemotherapy.

During surgery the bulk of the tumor is removed; however, there may still be a small microscopic tumor or tiny deposits of tumor cells left behind that were too small to have been detected and removed. After surgery the tumor will begin to grow again as the cancer cells

Starting Soon after Surgery

37

continue their normal dividing process. The smaller the tumor, the more rapid their growth. When the cancer is large, the percentage of cancer cells undergoing cell division decreases. If effective medications are applied to a small cancer, the chances of eliminating that cancer are much higher than if it is allowed to become very large and bulky because chemotherapy works most effectively on dividing cells. Therefore, it is most appropriate to use chemotherapy as soon after surgery as possible, when a large percent of the cancer cells are in the process of division.

Early use of the appropriate chemotherapeutic drugs can make the difference between a cure, temporary control, and no control at all. The importance and benefits of early treatment are illustrated in the following four case histories. The first two cases demonstrate the benefits of comprehensive and aggressive early treatment. The second two cases show the problems of delayed treatment.

Two Success Stories   A thirty-three year-old woman, the mother of four children ages one through nine, had one breast removed (a mastectomy) for breast cancer in December, 1976. Nine out of eighteen adjacent lymph nodes were involved with the cancer. Examinations that included X rays as well as liver and bone scans showed all else to be normal. Her estrogen-receptor level was 115 (anything above 10 is high). In order to reduce her estrogen supply, both her ovaries were removed. This was followed by chemotherapy with Cytoxan, Methotrexate and 5FU till 1978, and later she was given anti-estrogens. This patient, as of March, 1984, continued to be in excellent health without any return of the cancer (see facing photograph, taken in the summer of '84).

The next woman happens to be the best friend of the patient just described. She too had breast cancer, diagnosed in March, 1978, when she was thirty-five years old and had one daughter, ten years old. She had a mastectomy almost immediately. Her estrogen-receptor level was 37, and examination showed the cancer had spread to four out of eighteen nearby lymph nodes. She underwent nearly identical hormone and chemotherapy treatment as her friend, with the same gratifying results.

If these two patients had received no further treatment after the breast removals, a doctor's prediction of their futures would have been guarded. With four or more lymph nodes involved, there is a 90

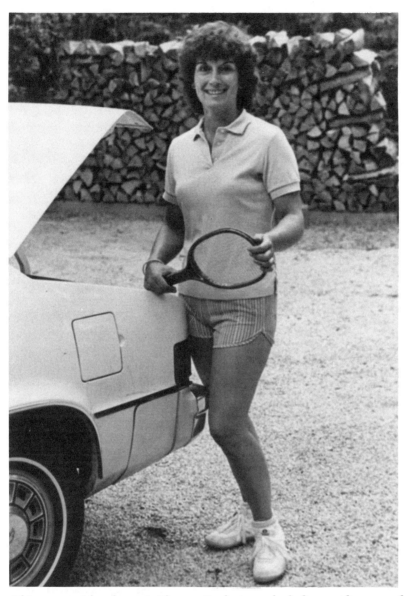

This woman (also shown in Chapter 1), photographed after an afternoon of racquetball, had a mastectomy, chemotherapy, and anti-estrogen treatment a few years ago. Today she's a healthy, skilled racquetball player who has won several league tournaments.

percent chance of a return of breast cancer within ten years. However, with aggressive hormone and chemotherapy treatment, these two close friends are alive and doing very well today. The results for the next two patients, who did not receive *early* aggressive treatment, are an entirely different matter.

A Case of Chemotherapy Not Started Soon
A sixty-four-year-old woman who had breast cancer had a mastectomy in April, 1974. It was discovered that only one out of twenty lymph nodes was involved with the tumor—but no further treatment was given to attack the cancer that had involved that one node. In March, 1976, she started having back and leg pains. By the time doctors could determine that the tumor had returned, she was bedridden with tumors all over her skin, lymph nodes and scalp, and practically all her bones were involved. A biopsy of a scalp tumor showed that the estrogen-receptor level was over 1,000, indicating the tumor was highly dependent on hormones to grow—a sign of a favorable outlook for her recovery.

The woman was started on chemotherapy and anti-hormones. Her initial response was quite dramatic, with all of the tumors in the skin, lymph nodes, and scalp disappearing completely. Furthermore, the bone tumor responded very well initially, although additional radiation was required to relieve pain in the pelvic area. Eventually a more potent combination of drugs was used, supplemented with the removal of the pituitary gland to eliminate the source of the hormone that the tumor depended upon to grow. She did quite well for two and a half years but eventually succumbed to the disease after about six more months. It is highly significant that this patient, who was completely bedridden prior to the chemotherapy and other forms of treatment, did so well for two and a half years.

On the other hand, this woman should have had a good chance for a much longer life because in 1974 she had only a very early involvement of the lymph system and also because the cancer was highly dependent on estrogen. Had she been started on chemotherapy and the anti-hormone drugs soon after her initial surgery, she would probably be alive today. (However, I should point out that this probability is not absolute fact.) Today, the choice of postsurgical treatments available for such a patient would, in most cases, automatically include aggressive chemotherapy plus anti-hormones, but the value of chemotherapy after surgery was not widely known in the early 1970s. Many of today's breast-cancer patients are now reaping the benefits of the intensive investigation and studies that took place in the second half of the '70s.

The second patient was a fifty-seven-year-old woman who was also diagnosed as having breast cancer, in this case in August, 1977. Six of nineteen lymph nodes were involved with tumors. Her doctor encouraged her to undergo chemotherapy, but she flatly refused because of her fear of the side effects of the drugs, having read negative literature on chemotherapy that a well-meaning friend had given her. She chose radiation therapy to the chest wall and did well until January, 1979, when she developed severe lower back pain and had great difficulty in walking. An investigation showed extensive tumor involvement in practically all her bones, especially in the spine. To prevent further damage to the spinal cord, additional radiation to the spine was given, but this time radiation was followed by chemotherapy plus anti-estrogens. She showed a dramatic improvement, regaining her ability to walk, and was able to go on several vacations from the Midwest to Florida and to the West Coast. In August, 1980, she developed neck pain and showed some cervical involvement. She received additional radiation to control the neck pain and was put on a different chemotherapeutic drug and another type of anti-estrogen. Even though she was not in complete remission she was still without symptoms in March, 1982, but she eventually succumbed to the disease.

Chemotherapy Postponed

Judging from this woman's marked response to treatment, it is safe to say that had she received chemotherapy soon after surgery, she would have responded considerably better, especially since the tumor at that time was much smaller. When the recurrence was discovered, she was once again not very receptive to the recommendations of her new oncologist. After considerable explanation (including a viewing of her bone scan), the patient changed her mind. Of the side effects she feared, one took place: she did eventually suffer complete (but only temporary) hair loss. Ironically, she did not lose her hair during her first chemotherapeutic combination—which is all she would have required with early treatment. And she experienced only slight nausea.

In cancer treatment more than any other field of medicine, the decisions that are made early in the course of the disease have a profound influence on the outcome. It is most disturbing to see a patient who, at the time of diagnosis, is advised by the family physician to go to an oncologist but has refused to do so because he or she is afraid of chemotherapy. Quite often the particular treatment is not as harsh as

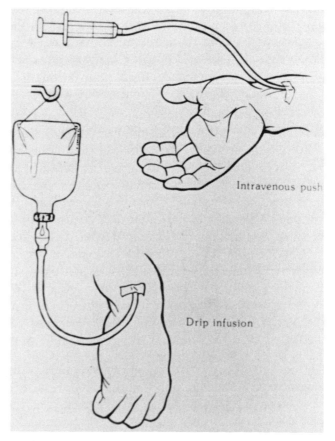

Two ways chemotherapeutic drugs are given. Which type to use in a particular case depends on both the tumor being treated and the properties of the drug being given.

imagined. Many of these patients finally do see an oncologist—but when the cancer is at a far advanced stage and the opportunity of a cure or long-term remission has become almost zero. *It is crucial that*

42

patients at least discuss the situation thoroughly with a specialist so they can make informed decisions.

In most cases chemotherapy is administered through the veins, either by a push or by drip infusion. However, these are often supplemented by oral medications or injections into the muscles, and occasionally chemotherapy is given through the artery that goes directly into the tumor. At times a combination of medications—four or even more—may be necessary to treat a single cancer, and occasionally not all medications will be given in the same way. Different methods of administration are used for different situations.

Ways Chemotherapy Is Given

An *intravenous (IV) push* is an injection into a vein. The decision to use the intravenous push depends on the type of tumor being treated and the chemicals that are effective against it, the most important factor being the physical and chemical properties of the medication. Some, such as nitrogen mustard, are stable only for about two minutes after they are mixed and must therefore be given rapidly. Injection into the vein is the only way to administer such a drug. Other medications—5FU and Methotrexate, for example—are mild; even in concentrated form they do not irritate the vein, so they too can be administered in a quick push (injection).

Medication to be given via the intravenous push is drawn into a syringe and pushed directly into the vein. The IV push is started with a small needle attached to three to five inches of tubing. When the needle is securely in place, the tubing is connected to a syringe containing the medication. The medication is pushed rapidly or slowly into the vein by the physician or nurse. An intravenous push usually takes only five to ten minutes and is often done in the doctor's office.

The Intravenous Push

An *intravenous drip infusion* is when medication is dripped slowly into the vein over a period of time ranging from about twenty minutes to over twenty-four hours. The drip infusion is chosen when the physical or chemical properties of a medication make the intravenous push undesirable. For example, the drugs may be too concen-

The Intravenous Drip Infusion

43

trated to be pushed directly into the vein and must be dissolved in additional fluid. If, for instance, a patient were given medications such as BCNU as a rapid intravenous push, the patient could experience some pain or burning and vein spasms. In other cases (though more rarely), when medications such as VP16 are given rapidly they can cause mild to moderate hypotension (low blood pressure), a problem easily corrected by slowing down the rate of speed with which the medicine goes into the vein. And a few medications are simply more effective when infused over several hours.

The infusion is started in the same way as an intravenous push, but this time a solution of sugar or salt water goes into the vein first, and when the solution is flowing well the chemotherapeutic drug is added to the bag of fluid. The flow is adjusted to the most desirable rate, which can be as short as twenty minutes or more than a day. Depending on the type of medication and the time required to administer it, the procedure can be done on an outpatient or inpatient basis. An infusion that takes less time can be done in a doctor's office.

Drip infusions bring us to the subject of financial realities. Whether the infusion is done in the doctor's office or in the hospital can depend not only on the complexity of the particular chemotherapy treatment but also on medical insurance. Some insurance policies simply do not cover this procedure adequately when it is done in the doctor's office—even though it may be much cheaper and easier that way. Some policies, unfortunately, do not cover this procedure at all when done in an office. It is not unusual for an insurance company to limit its payment to a sum that does not even cover the cost of the drugs—which can be as high as $200—let alone the cost of the doctor's or hospital's time. It is important to know your insurance coverage well in order to find ways of reducing the financial burden (see Chapter 8).

Intramuscular Injections

Intramuscular injections—injections into muscles—are usually given to supplement intravenous medications, but there are only a few drugs that can be administered by injection into muscles. Again, the main reason has to do with the characteristics of the medication. When intramuscular medications are used, they are only a part, but almost never all, of a patient's overall program. The injections are usually given in the buttocks on a weekly or monthly basis and can be done in a doctor's office.

44

Oral medications—given through the mouth—are sometimes used to supplement intravenous combination chemotherapy. Most chemotherapeutic drugs cannot be taken orally because the enzymes and chemicals of the body's digestive system will break down their chemical composition and render them inactive. In some instances, the drugs are simply not absorbed into the blood, and in other cases they may cause too much irritation to the stomach. In only a few situations will oral medications be sufficient to treat a particular type of cancer; among cancers that do qualify are chronic leukemias, bone-marrow tumors (multiple myeloma), prostate cancer, and breast cancer that has a very high estrogen receptor and occurs in elderly women.

When oral medications are necessary, they are usually taken for five to ten days each month. Occasionally they are taken daily for as long as the medication is effective. If side effects result, it would be because of the medication, not because it is taken orally.

Another method of administering chemotherapy is *intra-arterial perfusion*—injection directly into the artery—thereby delivering a large amount of medication directly to the tumor. (The difference between *per*fusion and *in*fusion is that perfusion is via the artery, while infusion is through the vein.)

Perfusion is particularly useful in *selected* patients with cancer of the colon that has spread to the liver. Perfusion can also be used for patients who have severe liver pain or patients whose tumors are principally limited to the liver and are not responding well to intravenous chemotherapy. Although this method of treatment can result in drastic improvement in a liver tumor, it must be stressed that perfusion is not recommended for most patients with liver metastasis; in fact, it is helpful to only a very small percentage of patients. For a patient to be selected for this procedure, the tumor must be primarily limited to the liver. Patients with liver tumors that have spread to other organs are generally not candidates for perfusion because it does not make sense to treat the liver only, when tumors are growing elsewhere.

Intra-arterial perfusion is also becoming increasingly useful in the treatment of brain tumors. Normally, drugs given intravenously are not effective on brain tumors because blood vessels in the brain possess a unique barrier that prevents foreign elements from entering the brain substance. However, if a large dose of medication is put directly into the neck artery that is carrying blood to the tumor, the barrier is overcome and the tumor is exposed to a substantial amount of the drug. This can lead to significant destruction of the tumor. While this method of treatment may not necessarily lead to a cure, it can cause a major reduction of the symptoms and a markedly improved quality of life for several months. But I must caution patients that not all brain or liver tumors respond to this method of treatment.

How Perfusion Is Given   Intra-arterial perfusion, whether to the liver or to the brain, is done while the patient is fully conscious; injections are given for sedation and to kill any pain. Then, with the patient under local anesthesia, a small incision is made and a flexible tube is placed in the major artery leading to the tumor. In order to pinpoint the specific route of the blood going directly to the tumor, a dye is injected (often causing a sensation of warmth throughout the patient's body), and the tube is carefully threaded into the pinpointed artery. When the tube is precisely positioned, the drugs can be infused at a steady, predetermined rate regulated by a portable pump. The drugs can either be given rapidly, and the tube removed, or the tube can be sutured in place and chemotherapy infused daily for several days, weeks, or even months in the patient's home with a portable pump.

CHAPTER SIX

Effects of Chemotherapy

Chemotherapy has two effects: the first is on the tumor itself and the second is on the body of the patient. The effect that chemotherapy does *not* have is magic; no single drug is effective against all types of cancer. The discovery of methods of curing or controlling cancer, like discoveries regarding the control of viruses, has been and continues to be a slow process. The common cold is caused by viruses—but there is no cure because no one medication is effective against all the different viruses that can cause colds, any more than the vaccine for polio can be effective against smallpox, chickenpox or measles.

I cannot overemphasize the fact that cancer is more than one disease; therefore, it is not likely that a single drug or treatment will ever be found that can control all of its variations. It is important to take with a grain of salt—maybe a whole pound of salt—any claims regarding the discovery of a miracle drug that is labelled *the* cure for cancer.

The effects of chemotherapy on cancer vary widely, depending on the type of drugs being used and the type of tumor being treated. Generally, the effects can be classified into five broad categories:

- Permanent remission: cure;
- Temporary remission: temporary control or temporary eradication of the tumor;

- Partial remission: significant reduction in the size or spread of the tumor;
- Stabilization: the tumor remaining the same, neither spreading nor shrinking;
- No improvement: insensitivity to chemotherapy.

Complete Remission

Many tumors can now be classified as curable. The first stage of a *cure* is complete eradication of the tumor: complete remission. When all of the *visible* tumor is destroyed, however, it does not necessarily mean that all the cancer cells have been destroyed.

Ridding a body of cancer is like ridding a garden of weeds—a conscientious gardener may spend hours pulling up unwanted plants, but if a shred of root or tuber remains in the garden, the dandelion, buttercup, chickweed, whatever, is likely to pop up again. With cancer, the unwanted growth may appear to the naked eye to have been completely weeded out, but in fact over 10 million cancer cells can still remain in the body—and these cells cannot be detected by any currently available tests or X rays. (As a yardstick of how tiny the cells are, a tumor about the size of a dime can contain about 1 billion cancer cells.)

Why Chemotherapy Must Be Continued

It is more difficult to wipe out the remaining cancer cells than to destroy the large tumor, which is why chemotherapy may be needed for a long period of time, even when the patient has apparently entered complete remission. If treatment is prematurely discontinued (that is, immediately after all of the visible tumor has disappeared), there is a great likelihood that the undetectable cancer cells will start growing again and become more resistant to subsequent medication. Many tumors that are now curable thus require prolonged treatment ranging anywhere from eight months to three years. The time required for chemotherapy to produce a complete cure depends on the particular tumor. Chemotherapy for, say, six to nine months may result in a cure for Hodgkin's disease, for example, while about three years of intensive treatment at various intervals may be required to produce a complete cure in some forms of acute lymphoblastic leukemia. The interval between complete remission and the point where the patient can be declared cured

48

depends, again, on the particular tumor. A patient who has a testicular tumor and been in complete remission for only two years after chemotherapy is very likely to be considered in permanent remission and cured.

Temporary remission means that although the tumor at one time appeared to have been eradicated, after a period of time it can again be seen or felt. In many instances, if the tumor, after treatment, has not reappeared after two or three years or more, the chances of its reappearing are slim. *Temporary Remission*

However, there are certain tumors (for example, breast cancer) that can come back even twenty years after surgery. It is comforting to know, though, that the longer the tumor is kept under control the less likely it is to return. Furthermore, the longer the tumor is kept in remission before it reappears, the more likely that it can be controlled after a second or sometimes even a third course of treatment. Ideally, of course, the tumor will be controlled the first time around. It is often difficult for patients who are doing very well, without any evidence of a tumor, to understand why they should continue with treatment. However, considering that as many as 10 million cancer cells can go completely undetected, attempts should be made to eliminate as many abnormal cells as possible in order to produce long-term remission or cure.

Partial remission means that there has been some reduction in the tumor's size even though it may not have completely disappeared. At this stage, many patients can resume normal activity. The duration of a partial remission—the amount of time before the tumor begins to grow again—varies widely. When treatment is resumed, a different set of medications may be used, with some additional response. However, a partial response at this point is not a very favorable sign since there must be a complete response in order to achieve a cure. *Partial Remission*

In many cases chemotherapy does not significantly reduce the tumor's size but may have the effect of *stabilizing the disease*, preventing it from growing any larger or spreading. If it is possible to stabilize a tumor that is not causing any significant problems, the *Stabilization*

49

patient can continue normal activity until the tumor starts growing out of control. Quite often, if a tumor is stabilized, other types of medication can be used to attempt to produce a better response.

The reason why some cancer cells, after being controlled or stabilized, start growing again is that they have developed resistance to the medications. Resistance can occur when the outer coatings of cancer cells develop changes that prevent the chemicals from penetrating the cells. In addition, cancer cells can also develop new enzymes that can neutralize a drug or repair drug-induced damage.

Reducing
Tumor-cell Resistance

Tumor cells are most likely to become resistant to chemotherapy when only one drug is used at a time; thus, by using several drugs at once, this tendency can be reduced. It is less likely that the cancer cells will be able to develop an immunity to all the different drugs that are used in a combination. (As with all rules, there are exceptions to the several-drugs-at-once rule: In the treatment of chronic leukemias or bone tumors (myeloma) a single drug used at intervals can keep the cancer under control for three to five years or even more.)

When different drugs are used simultaneously (usually two, three, or four different types), each attacks the cancer cells from a different angle; consequently, combination chemotherapy produces the most dramatic effects on the disease. Equally important is the fact that when several drugs are used at once, none has to be given in an extremely high dose, so the result is that side effects are minimized. In the treatment of Hodgkin's disease, for example, five different medications can be used at the same time. Of these, three important ones have no adverse effects whatsoever on the bone marrow, where the blood cells are formed, so they do not result in the common side effect of a lowered blood count.

Tumors
That Do Not Respond
To Chemotherapy

Some tumors show complete *insensitivity* to chemotherapy. Treatment of such tumors, even if given at the earliest sign of spread, does not seem to offer any significant benefit. There are two choices for the patient in this situation: either not to take any more treatment or to go to a research institute for treatment with experimental drugs. In using experimental drugs, scientists often have a very good idea of what kind of response to expect with cancers that are insensitive to the more usual treatments. However, if a cancer does not respond to experimental drugs, it is often better to discontinue additional treatment and let the patient lead as normal a life as possible.

This was the decision in the case of a particularly pleasant twenty-nine-year-old man, the father of three young children, whom I came to know when he was found to have cancer on his chest wall. The cancer had spread from a black pigment on his skin. When the man was diagnosed, in March of 1980, no spread was noted and he was appropriately treated with surgery alone. Three months later, he had a rapidly-developing node larger than an egg in the left armpit. This was surgically removed and a complete examination showed that it was the same tumor, which had spread from the chest wall. No further spread was noted.

No effective chemotherapy exists for this type of cancer and the experimental drugs used on this specific disease are rather harsh. The oncologist, in consulting with other experts, all with a special interest in this particular cancer, decided that the most prudent approach was simply observation, without any radiation or chemotherapy. A major factor in the decision to suspend treatment was the fact that this type of cancer is very unpredictable and can lie dormant for months or even years before starting another rapid growth. Fortunately, the patient, when last seen in March, 1984, continued to be free of disease. Deciding to withhold treatment is very unusual and is contrary to the typical recommendation of attacking as soon as possible any cancer that has spread. However, the patient in this case is in excellent health and three years after the second surgery was working full time without any evidence of the disease. The "treatment" plan here underscores the critical need for the physicians involved to be thoroughly familiar with various types of cancer and to treat each patient as an individual.

An Unusual Decision: Observation, Not Treatment

The most well-known side effect of chemotherapy is nausea and vomiting. The fact is, although some chemotherapeutic drugs can cause violent reactions, others do not result in any nausea or

Side Effects: Nausea and Vomiting

vomiting at all. It is simply a matter of which drugs are being used and how large the dose is—in general, the larger the dose, the more likely the possibility of nausea.

Psychological Considerations

The patient's psychological state can drastically ease or worsen this particular side effect of chemotherapy. One patient I know of, a man with leukemia, never—not even once—got sick during chemotherapy even though he received at least ten chemicals, some of which make almost every patient ill. At times he would have a very large dose of medication and be on a plane the same afternoon or the next day on a business trip. Such toughness (and luck) may be unique, but the story is worth telling.

On the other hand, some patients are afflicted with nausea before the treatment starts, and in one case a sixty-four-year-old man developed problems because of a conversation with another patient. The older man had cancer of the lymph system and had tolerated his treatment extremely well for about eight months, but one day he talked to a patient who went into minute detail about how chemotherapy always made him sick. After that the patient began getting nauseated and vomiting even before his treatments. During one of the area's worst blizzards, the patient was in the hospital for chemotherapy but his oncologist was unable to make it. The next day when the patient saw his physician, he described how sick he got promptly at 9:00 a.m. (his usual treatment time) even though no chemotherapy was administered.

All this really means, of course, is that everyone reacts differently to chemotherapy. There's no denying that certain drugs are likely to cause nausea—but there are always patients who surprise medical science. In any case, most people simply react according to their own bodily and psychological chemistry, for better or worse. Bear in mind that *only a small percentage of patients have severe nausea and vomiting as a side effect of chemotherapy.*

Anti-nausea Treatment

Fortunately, regardless of the cause, nausea and vomiting can be minimized. When the medication causes discomfort and the reaction is a minor queasy feeling, anti-nausea medications given orally prior to treatment and taken at various intervals during the first day after treatment can be of considerable help. These drugs cannot offer much benefit if the patient is already throwing up, of course, since the anti-nausea medicine would be vomited up along with everything else. A patient in this situation might benefit from anti-nausea medication given as a suppository. Another solution—if a spouse, other family member or neighbor can do so—would be intramuscular injections of anti-nausea medicine given at home. In severe cases it may be advisable to admit the patient to the hospital so that the anti-nausea drug can be given overnight with intramuscular (IM) or intravenous (IV) injections. Occasionally, if a very large amount of chemotherapeutic drugs must be given, the amount can be divided in order to reduce the side effects of a single strong dose at one time. Psychiatric or psychological help, including hypnosis, has been effective to some extent in controlling nausea due to emotional factors.

It is important to remember that in most instances short-term nausea and vomiting are not a large price to pay for the potentially long-term control or possible cure of cancer.

Hair Loss Although loss of hair is another common problem, I should stress that significant hair loss, like nausea, happens with only a small percent of patients. The extent of hair loss resulting from chemotherapy varies widely, depending on the type of medications and, especially, on whether or not the patient has received two or more medications that each tend to produce this side effect. The majority of medications cause either no hair loss at all or just a small amount of loss—a thinning that is scarcely noticeable. Quite often the patient may lose a small amount of hair over the first few months, then find that the loss has stopped and in fact that the hair is starting to grow again—even though the patient may still be on chemotherapy. Most women on mild to strong chemotherapy are able, if they want, to have permanents, since their hair loss is not significant.

There are some medications that, if used alone, produce a small to moderate amount of hair loss but which, when used in combination with other medications, produce complete hair loss. When Adriamycin and Oncovin are combined, the hair loss is usually total and usually happens within two to three weeks. Since the degree of hair loss is predictable once the type of drug and treatment are determined, the oncologist may suggest that wig be purchased in advance.

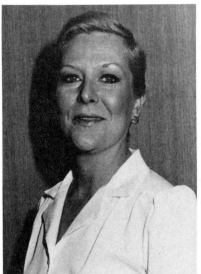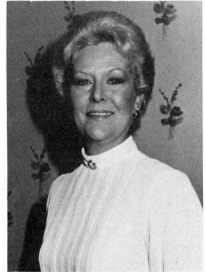

Although this patient lost all her hair while receiving Adriamycin and Oncovin, the hair started growing back when she was switched to CMF, another drug combination. The photo at right shows her on the last day of her CMF chemotherapy, hair completely regrown.

Unexpected Hair Loss   Hair loss has been known to occur at the most inopportune moments and without warning. I know of a young businessman who was undergoing many cycles of chemotherapy for leukemia and at one point had lost all his hair, which had fully regrown. During a subsequent course of Adriamycin and Oncovin treatment, he lost his hair suddenly, and reported this incident to his doctor: "A funny thing happened to me last week when I went to Washington for a seminar. When I got off the plane, a strong wind was blowing and all my hair fell out except for a small tuft on top. I felt like joining a Hare Krishna group but instead went to a wig shop, purchased a wig and went off to my seminar with new hair." This particular patient tolerated his prolonged treatment especially well partly because of his determination to carry on, no matter what. Being able to hang onto a sense of humor in such circumstances is a great advantage.

The loss of hair is *not* a permanent condition, and after chemotherapy is finished (or sometimes even before), the hair will start growing back. By the end of treatment the hair can be as full and luxuriant as ever, although once in a while there may be a slight change in texture or color.

A decrease of blood cells is one of the most common, and a very significant, side effect of chemotherapy. Probably over 80 percent of the chemotherapeutic drugs lower the blood count—how much depends upon the dose and the type of medication. It is particularly important to understand the significance of this side effect in order to cooperate with the oncologist as much as possible to minimize any potentially serious complications.

The human body contains three major groups of blood cells: white, red, and platelets. These cells are made on the inside of the bone in the marrow, especially in the skull, spine, hips and breastbone (the sternum, which supports most of the ribs as well as collarbone). It takes about five to ten days for these cells to be manufactured. From the marrow they are carried to the bloodstream to do their work.

There are many different types of *white cells*, but the basic function of all of them is to fight infection. A normal white-cell count is 4,000 to 7,000, which would show up as 4.0 to 7.0 on a hospital's computer printout. (Hospitals being no different from the rest of the world, medical information these days is frequently stated in terms mandated by computers). If the white count drops below 1,000 (1.0), particularly to around 500 (.5), the chances of the patient getting a serious infection are markedly increased. The patient with a very low white count is likely to have a fever even if there is no infection. When a white count drops to around 400 (.4), the physician will usually have the patient admitted to the hospital. As soon as a patient develops a fever, blood, throat and urine cultures are taken to try to see if an infection exists and, if it does, to find its source. The patient is usually put on two or three very strong antibiotics while waiting for the results of the tests. If an infection is found, the patient continues on the antibiotics for ten to fourteen days. If no infection is found after about five days, then the fever is probably due

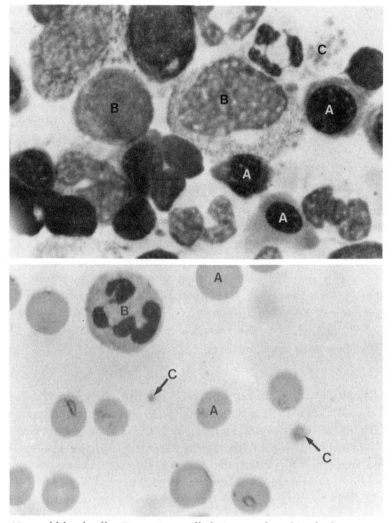

Normal blood cells. *Top:* young cells being produced in the bone marrow. *Bottom:* mature cells in the blood. *A* indicates red cells; *B*, white cells; *C*, platelets.

to the low white count itself, and the antibiotics are then discontinued. When a patient is not in the hospital, it is absolutely necessary for the family to call the oncologist if a fever develops, especially with chills, no matter what the time, day or night. Do not wait and say, "I think it's going to go away." Unless the infection is very unusual, it can be attacked by antibiotics that now can cure most types of infection. In cancer patients with very low blood count, it is urgent to treat the infection early. To some degree these patients already have low resistance; because of the absence of the infection-fighting white cells, any infectious organisms can multiply unchecked very rapidly, with serious consequences. Antibiotics given early can often keep the infections under control until the white blood cells recover to destroy the infections.

The major function of the *red cells* is to carry oxygen, via the *Red Cells* bloodstream, from the lungs to the body tissues. If the red-blood-cell count is low, the patient has anemia; the patient will have a low supply of oxygen, will look pale and will feel weak and fatigued, with shortness of breath. Fortunately, most chemotherapeutic drugs do not affect the red cells as much as they do the white cells and the platelets.

Platelets are tiny particles in the blood that stop or prevent *Platelets* bleeding by clotting at the site of an open injury such as a cut. If the platelets are low, the patient will have a tendency to bruise easily or to bleed from the gums or the nose. The severity of the bleeding depends upon how low the platelet count is. The normal platelet count varies from between 150,000 to 400,000. Usually there is no serious bleeding unless the platelet count is lower than 15,000 to 20,000. The major warning sign of a low platelet count is a skin rash in which tiny bleeding spots—petechiae—appear on the skin. Another sign is black and blue marks: bruises or, more technically, ecchymoses. Again, it is very important to call the oncologist as soon as any bleeding spots, bruises or any other form of bleeding appears during chemotherapy.

White cells normally live for about two days and then die. *Replacement* Platelets live for about nine days and red cells, for about one hun- *of Blood Cells* dred and twenty. Since the lifespan of these cells is short, they must be manufactured through cell division, at a rapid rate, in order to replace those that are dying off. This fast division of blood cells explains why they are affected by chemotherapy: The medicines in-

57

terfere with any kind of rapid cell division, including that which is normal and necessary. Fortunately, one characteristic of blood cells is their great ability to reproduce; consequently, the damaging effect of chemotherapy on these cells is temporary. If the blood count is low as a result of chemotherapy, there is very little a patient can do to make the count increase. Taking iron or vitamins, resting or getting fresh air, probably will not make much difference unless the patient has a specific nutritional deficiency. One thing that can be done, and is easy, is to replace both the red cells and platelets by transfusion. So far, no very effective means has been devised for replacing white cells, but researchers appear to be getting close to solving the problem, and the medical community is hopeful that it will soon be as easy to replace white cells as red cells and platelets.

If the blood count is low when the patient is due for treatment, treatment may be delayed until the blood count has improved. If the blood count is not extremely low, the dose of the medication can simply be adjusted so that the blood count is not in danger of dropping too far. I should point out that in most cases the blood count doesn't give any indication as to what the patient's tumor is doing—it only gives information to determine whether or not to give additional chemotherapy at a particular time or whether to adjust the dose. There is no reason at all for a patient to become upset because the blood count is low (although the complications of low blood count—fever, for example—may sometimes be frightening). As for the effects of low blood count on treatment: in only a very small number of cases will patients require major adjustments in chemotherapy because of low blood counts. The number is even smaller for those who might require hospitalization for transfusions or special treatment for low counts.

Sore Mouth or Throat   Another place where cells are dividing at a rapid rate is in the digestive system—all the way from the throat to the intestines. Many cells in the digestive tract are replaced every three days, so there must be rapid division in order for these cells to replace the ones that have been sloughed off. The effect of chemotherapy on these rapidly dividing cells is the reason why a patient might develop a sore mouth or throat or, occasionally, bowel problems.

The soreness can be successfully treated by medications

58

specifically manufactured for the mouth and throat—anesthetic suspensions and/or antibiotics, since mouth sores can become infected. Often the throat is infected with a particular fungus known as candida. This can be treated with mycostatin suspension, which is very effective against candida, and patients using it often show a dramatic improvement. These measures for severe sore throat may cause the side effects to disappear in a few days. In cases when the soreness takes the form of small ulcers in the mouth, the treatment is the same.

In any case, good oral hygiene is essential for anyone on chemotherapy. On many occasions the severity of the sore throat parallels the severity of a low white-cell count, and the situation often starts improving as soon as the white count starts going up. Since a severe sore throat and a severe low white-cell count may go hand in hand, severe throat problems should be reported to the oncologist as soon as possible.

Bowel Problems

Although acute diarrhea can sometimes be associated with chemotherapy, the condition is usually short-lived and often does not require treament.

The opposite condition—constipation—is far more likely to occur. Major reasons for this are inactivity on the part of the patient and heavy doses of pain killers (particularly narcotics), which, like chemotherapeutic drugs such as Oncovin or Velban, can result in constipation. Sometimes constipation may be severe enough to cause impaction, which is a hard stool high up in the rectum that is very difficult to evacuate. Often impaction requires the manual breaking up of the stool and the use of enemas afterward.

Constipation can be avoided by a routine use of stool softeners or bulk laxatives. If these preventive measures are not successful, the use of stronger laxatives and enemas should be started at once because severe constipation is a painful and exhausting experience.

As with all side effects, a patient should discuss bowel problems with the oncologist immediately.

Muscle Problems

Some medications can cause muscle weakness, occasional muscular cramps, or numbness and tingling in the fingertips. If the symptoms are severe, the medication that is responsible can be reduced or temporarily discontinued, but in most instances the symptoms are just a nuisance and not severe enough to warrant reducing or stopping the therapy.

General Side Effects   Some general side effects of chemotherapy include weakness, fatigue, dizziness, dehydration and changes in weight. Weakness and fatigue may be direct results of the medication and can last one or two days after each treatment. Weakness along with dizziness could also be experienced by patients whose chemotherapy causes severe nausea and vomiting. These same patients may experience slight to moderate dehydration. The length of this side effect can be shortened considerably by intravenous hydration given in the hospital overnight, or on an outpatient basis, or at home. (Many home-care agencies can give IV's at patients' homes.) Since dizziness could also be due to low blood cells or could be a direct effect of the tumor, any persistent dizziness should be brought to the doctor's attention.

Sometimes a patient's weight will change during chemotherapy. If the patient loses weight, and the loss is temporary, it is the result of nausea and vomiting. Persistent weight loss is the result of the tumor. Weight gain, however, is probably more common than weight loss for patients on chemotherapy. Sometimes this may be a direct effect of the medication, especially in patients on hormones such as cortisone or female hormones such as DES. More often, though, weight gain is due to anxiety, which is accompanied by persistent nibbling. Moderate exercise and involvment in activities that take the patient's mind away from the illness can prevent excessive eating.

Concerns about Fertility   The testes and ovaries produce cells that divide at a moderately rapid rate—the cells of the sperm and the eggs. About 80 percent of women who are of menstruating age and are placed on chemotherapy for breast cancer will stop menstruating. For some, it may be a matter of several months before they resume their periods after chemotherapy has ended. And in men the sperm count may drop considerably. This does not necessarily mean that men and women who receive chemotherapy will not be able to have children.

For a man in chemotherapy the sperm count is usually extremely low, so the chances of reproduction are very small during treatment. It may take several months or years before the sperm count returns to nearly normal. Some authorities have advised that patients store sperm at sperm banks prior to chemotherapy, but there is no study showing how successful these sperm will be in producing pregnancies.

In women, the story is a little bit different. Depending upon the age of the patient and the amount of chemotherapy, treatment could result in the ovaries not producing eggs. The older the patient, the more likely this is to happen, and the less the amount of drug required to produce this effect. This may lead to decreased libido (interest in sex) and the irregular and infrequent menstrual periods that signal the onset of menopause. In other words, the older the patient, and the greater the dose of chemotherapeutic drugs, the greater the possibility that the woman's menopause will start early. In any case, it is imperative that a woman avoid pregnancy while taking any drug that affects rapidly dividing cells (which means all chemotherapeutic drugs).

Necessity for Avoiding Pregnancy

Some chemotherapeutic medications, such as Methotrexate, are known specifically to cause abortions or deformed fetuses, but *many* chemotherapeutic drugs could be so damaging that pregnancy must be postponed. As for the length of the postponement: No one knows how long to advise a woman to wait after chemotherapy before she starts attempting to have children. Many experts would honestly say they have no way of answering this question, since there are no complete data on this issue. Some oncologists advise patients to wait until they have been in remission two to three years before trying to conceive, which allows time to see whether the remission will continue. It is not known what long-term effects the cancer-killing chemicals might eventually have on the babies born to cancer patients, but so far many of the babies appear to be as healthy as any other children. A few very small studies of women in remission have indicated some slight chances of adverse outcomes of pregnancy such as spontaneous abortions or fetal abnormalities. But more recent larger studies revealed no fetal defects or abnormal outcomes of pregnancy. The fact is that adequate studies have not yet been done to answer the important questions regarding long-term effects of chemotherapy on reproduction. Only one thing is clear: a woman should avoid pregnancy while receiving chemotherapy.

Possible Second
Malignancy

The possibility of a second malignancy occurring as a result of chemotherapy is a question that is raised in medical circles but, practically speaking, this possibility should not be a deterrent to taking chemotherapy.

It is true that certain kinds of medications have produced or have been associated with leukemia in patients treated for cancer of the ovary or for bone tumors. In most of these situations the treatment was prolonged—over three to four years—and in other instances the patients received high doses of radiation in addition to chemotherapy. It is not absolutely clear whether the chemotherapy was the cause of these leukemias, or whether these particular cancer patients would tend to have more than one type of cancer regardless of chemotherapy. The important point is that patients should not receive chemotherapy unless they absolutely need it, and they should not receive it any longer than necessary. In many situations, it is not obvious how long treatment should last, so the question of length of treatment, which may have some influence on the development of a second tumor, is not easy to answer.

Clearly, though, the possibility of developing a second malignancy due to chemotherapy is extremely small. There are many patients whose life expectancy, without chemotherapy, would be measured in terms of only months or a few years at best, but who can be cured if chemotherapy is given. The consequences of not receiving chemotherapy are, in many instances, not only devastating, but often immediate. Nevertheless, every effort should of course be made to use these drugs judiciously.

Drugs That Ease
Side Effects

Many patients are reluctant to undergo chemotherapy because of their fear of the side effects. Thanks to recent research, such fear is often unwarranted; effective treatments have been developed to counteract various side effects, and more are on the way. An example is the case of Cisplatinum. Cisplatinum is one of the most effective chemotherapy drugs, but it causes such severe nausea and

62

vomiting that many patients are simply unable to take it even though their cancer may be potentially curable with Cisplatinum as the major drug in a combination. Recently, however, through use of various combinations of anti-nausea medications, the majority of patients have been able to take Cisplatinum with very little or no vomiting at all. This is a really significant step forward, since many chemotherapeutic medications become much more effective when used in combination with Cisplatinum.

As far as the general public is concerned, probably the best-publicized drug for reducing chemotherapeutically induced nausea is marijuana. Actually, it's one of the components of marijuana that has this effect—THC—and a number of studies have shown this chemical to be effective. But THC should not be looked upon as a cure-all, and should be taken with great care. It is available by prescription in pill form in several states, but its absorption rate into the blood stream is unpredictable, which probably explains the wide variation of success rates with patients. The pills have their own side effects such as hallucination, lack of coordination, fainting spells, and low blood pressure accompanied by dizziness. Of any group of patients taking the pills, from 5 to 35 percent will experience the side effects.

It has been argued that marijuana, when smoked, gets into the patient's system almost immediately, so that it not only takes effect right away but can be adjusted quickly for a larger or smaller dose.

Patients who ask their doctors about this might have difficulty getting answers, or getting THC, especially at small or community hospitals. At major cancer centers, however, it's easier to get marijuana pills. Marijuana as an anti-nausea medication has steadily lost its appeal to many physicians who used to prescribe it. There are more effective and safer methods of control than marijuana. In any case, marijuana does not work for everyone, and should only be used by carefully selected patients. Especially for the elderly it tends to be unsuccessful—although younger patients could see it as a bit of silver lining to their illness.

Improved control of the side effects of chemotherapy should be, and I believe will be, one of the primary goals of cancer researchers for the next few years. Success will not only make chemotherapy much easier but will also allow oncologists to prescribe higher doses of medication and get better results. There is a very good possibility that medications that relieve some of the problem side effects will become available in the near future.

Side Effects That Require Calling the Doctor It is important to call the doctor immediately if you experience any of the serious side effects described in this chapter. Here, in summary, are some side effects a doctor should be made aware of.

- Fever with a temperature over 101° or a very low temperature—about 95°;
- A very sore throat or mouth, or ulcers in the throat or mouth;
- Profuse sweating or chills strong enough to cause shaking;
- Dizziness, lethargy, or shortness of breath;
- A severe cold or flu (do not discount the importance of these; the physician may decide to delay the next chemotherapy treatment because of a severe cold);
- Bruises or tiny bleeding spots on the skin;
- Severe nausea and/or vomiting;
- Severe constipation or diarrhea;
- Marked pain or inflammation of the arm in which the chemotherapy was given;
- Severe headaches or *any* severe pain. These may not be the result of chemotherapy, but they could give a doctor useful information.

Any of these symptoms should be considered important, and any one of them requires that the physician be notified immediately.

CHAPTER SEVEN

Several Types of Cancer and Their Chemotherapy

This chapter deals with several types of cancer as well as their rates of cure, the numbers of people they afflict, those most likely to develop them, symptoms, and diagnosis. Rather than detailing information regarding the surgery or radiation that might be required for some of them, I have concentrated on chemotherapy only, since chemotherapy varies widely according to the cancer involved. Surgery and radiation, which are much less variable, are covered in detail in Chapter 4. In order to link real people to the technical information, I have concluded most sections with one or two case histories.

A simplified definition of *leukemia* would be: *any of several diseases involving uncontrolled proliferation of white blood cells.* It afflicts every age group and both sexes.

Leukemia

The diagnosis of leukemia is often very simple: a complete blood count is made and the blood cells are examined under a microscope. The diagnosis is confirmed by bone-marrow tests. When there is the slightest doubt about the exact diagnosis, the oncologist will usually consult with other specialists who have extensive experience in the diagnosis and treatment of leukemias.

Chronic Leukemia   There are over ten major types of leukemia; some are chronic and others are acute. The *chronic leukemias* progress slowly, usually not causing much in the way of problems for two or three years—even up to ten years in a few cases—many of them, in fact, not even requiring treatment for several years after diagnosis. No noticeable symptoms

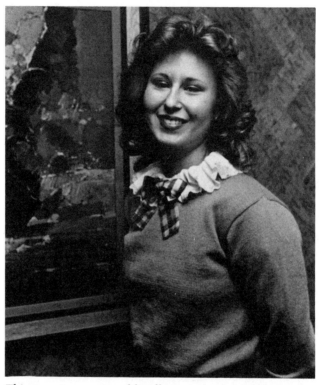

This twenty-one-year-old college senior was diagnosed at age thirteen with acute lymphoblastic leukemia (ALL), which once was almost always fatal. Her initial treatment was at a community hospital in consultation with a pediatric oncologist, followed by more intensive therapy at a teaching hospital. She is now in complete remission and probably cured. Although she bought a wig before her chemotherapy, she was one of the cases where a wig turned out to be unnecessary.

exist at the time of diagnosis in most chronic leukemias. They are often detected in routine checkups or during testing prior to entering the hospital for something else. A patient can have 100,000 white blood cells (a normal count is up to 10,000) without any problems. At an advanced stage, however, a patient may have fatigue, weight loss, excessive sweating, fever, may bruise easily and have a fullness in the abdomen due to a massively enlarged spleen. In cases of chronic lymphatic leukemia, enlarged lymph nodes often exist throughout the body. While there is no sure cure for chronic forms of leukemia, in most instances they can be treated and controlled with mild oral medications so that patients can lead normal, active lives for many years.

Acute leukemias are a different story. They are called "acute" because they progress rapidly and, if untreated, are quickly fatal. Of the acute leukemias, the one for which treatment has made the greatest progress, and whose cure rates have increased most significantly, is acute lymphoblastic leukemia (ALL), especially that of children. ("Lymphoblastic" refers to immature white blood cells formed in the bone marrow and lymph tissue.) Four thousand new cases of acute lymphoblastic leukemia in children are diagnosed every year in the United States, many of them in children between the ages of three and five. Prior to adequate chemotherapy, the majority of these children died of the disease within two months from the time of initial diagnosis, even though the diagnosis may have been made reasonably early (that is, within one month of the appearance of the symptoms).

Acute Leukemia

The symptoms of acute leukemia are usually due to the fact that cancer cells are replacing normal blood cells. Because of low counts of red and normal white blood cells and platelets, the patient will have symptoms of anemia, infection and various degrees of bleeding. Often bone pain or arthritis show up, especially in children.

So much progress has been made in the treatment of acute lymphoblastic leukemia that it is now possible to predict with great accuracy which patients with various types of this leukemia will respond best to treatment. For 60 percent of all children who have the disease, the outlook is favorable. Approximately 95 to 100 percent of the children in this *favorable* group will enter complete remission, and probably 75 percent of them will be cured completely. This is a significant improvement. While the treatment for adults with the same type of leukemia is not as successful, steady progress is definitely being made in the treatment of the adult type. The disease in adults seems to be more aggressive than it is in children—in fact, the younger the patient, the better the prognosis; children between the ages of two and ten respond more favorably than those who are older.

Necessary Treatment:
Chemotherapy

The only effective kind of treatment for any leukemia is chemotherapy. Since the disease is throughout the body, there is no specific area that can be pinpointed for attack, and both surgery and radiation are out of the question (although they may be used sometimes to provide relief from the pressure of a tumor).

Recent studies of the treatment of various leukemias have shown some very encouraging results in cases where the approach was aggressive but with careful monitoring. If chemotherapeutic drugs are given one at a time for ALL, the rate of success varies between 20 and 50 percent and usually lasts for only about three months. For example (in ALL), Oncovin produces a complete response in 40 percent of the cases, Prednisone in 35 percent, Adriamycin in 45 percent. However, if all three drugs are used together, the result is complete remission in 75 to 100 percent of the patients. The problem now is to keep the patient in complete remission once the combination of the three drugs has eliminated the cancer. From about 1981, various combinations of up to ten different chemicals have produced an even greater percentage of long-term, complete responses. Side effects of the treatment, obviously, depend on the medications used.

One Example of
Successful Treatment

An example of a complete response produced by the aggressive use of chemotherapy with careful monitoring of the side effects can be illustrated by the following case.

In December, 1978, around Christmastime, a thirty-six-year-old father of five came to the hospital because he had a fever and anemia so severe that he required transfusions. Examination revealed that he had an enlarged spleen and liver as well as numerous enlarged lymph nodes throughout his body. His bone marrow was packed with leukemia cells that had completely replaced all the normal cells. The diagnosis of acute lymphoblastic leukemia was made and the man was started on chemotherapy. After three days his white-blood-cell count dropped from 4,500 to

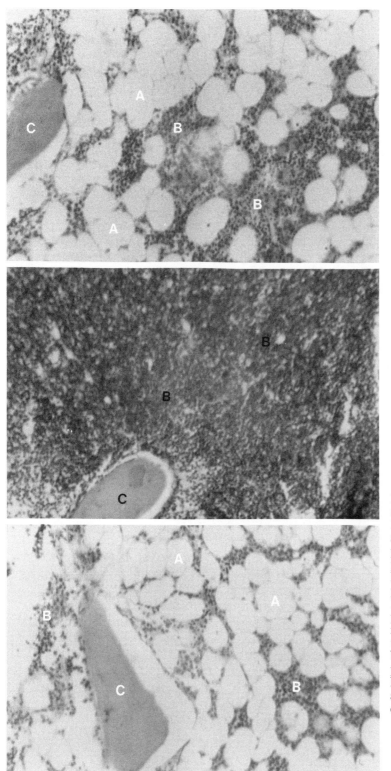

Effectiveness of combination chemotherapy in leukemia. Normal bone marrow (top and bottom) consists of 50 percent fat clusters (A) and 50 percent blood cells (B). C is hard bone. In the middle photo, taken in December 1978, leukemia cells have replaced the entire bone marrow. The bottom picture, taken in February, 1980, is bone marrow from the same patient. The leukemia cells have completely disappeared, and fat clusters and normal cells have reappeared.

600, at which time he developed an infection, but this was only a minor problem and was easily treated. Within a week all visible evidence of leukemia had disappeared. The patient tolerated his treatment remarkably well, the only side effects being temporary hair loss and an excessive appetite whenever Prednisone was given. Nausea and vomiting were barely a problem, even in over eighteen months of treatment. Because side effects were minimal and because treatment (intravenous chemotherapy) was given before or after work hours, this man has been able to lead a full and active life. He has rarely missed a day's work and was still in complete remission in March, 1984, the last time I saw him.

The prognosis for treatment of leukemia is promising, especially with some forms of acute lymphoblastic childhood leukemia. In other types, and in acute leukemias in adults, the present outlook is one of guarded optimism.

Hodgkin's Disease   *Hodgkin's disease* is a form of cancer of the lymph glands. Today over 70 percent of the patients with advanced Hodgkin's disease, if treated with chemotherapy, attain complete remission lasting over ten years (meaning they appear to be cured); if the disease is treated in an early stage, 90 percent of the patients can be cured with radiation alone. Although it comprises only 1 percent of all new cancers, Hodgkin's disease is important because of its economic and social impact, due to the age of those developing it. This cancer usually afflicts people either in their late teens to early thirties or between the ages of forty-five and fifty—in other words, people in the prime of life and in their most productive years.

Because the disease is a cancer of the lymph glands, its major symptoms are lumps in the neck region, under the armpits, or in the groin. In many instances patients have no symptoms; however, when the disease is more advanced, patients may complain of profuse night sweats, fever, significant weight loss or itchy skin. Diagnosis is often suspected during a routine chest X ray when enlarged lymph nodes are found. Otherwise, diagnosis is made by a biopsy of the involved tissue (usually any readily accessible lymph nodes).

The extent, or staging, of the disease is an important aspect of treatment planning. The staging of Hodgkin's disease is as follows:

Stage 1: only one lymph-node area is involved;

Stage 2: two or more lymph-node areas are involved on the same side of the diaphragm;

Stage 3: two or more lymph-node areas are involved on different sides of the diaphragm, but no vital organs are involved;

Stage 4: vital organs such as the bone marrow, lung, liver and brain are involved.

Early stages (1 and 2) can be treated with radiation alone, whereas advanced stages (3 and 4) are treated with chemotherapy with or without radiation. The standard chemotherapy treatment is called MOPP (an abbreviation of four drugs: nitrogen mustard, Oncovin, Procarbazine and Prednisone) and is very effective, resulting in long-term remission and survival. If the disease does return, it usually does so within the first two years after the treatment has ended. Only very rarely does Hodgkin's disease come back after five years. In fact, the longer the interval of complete remission, the greater the likelihood that even if the disease does come back it can be treated with a great chance of achieving a second, complete remission. Treatment for Hodgkin's disease is so well standardized that it is easily available for all competent oncologists in an average community hospital. The treatment program I have outlined here is slightly oversimplified, and treatment will vary in some cases.

It must be pointed out that the chemotherapy for Hodgkin's disease is one of the most difficult treatments for cancer patients because the drugs cause severe nausea and vomiting, which can last up to four or six hours. There may also be significant hair loss, numbness and tingling in the fingers and, occasionally, severe weakness of the legs. The other side effect may be severe constipation due to Oncovin, especially during the first two months of treatment. There are established ways to treat constipation in order to minimize the discomfort. It is important for patients to persevere and complete their treatment because the potential of complete cure is so great that the sacrifice is well worth it.

The importance of determining the stage of the disease and thus *Two Successes* the appropriate treatment is illustrated by the case of a thirty-year-old woman who had a neck lump that was biopsied. An oncologist and a pathologist viewed the slides from the biopsy independently and both came to the same conclusion: Hodgkin's disease. An X ray showed a large mass in the chest, and the patient was tentatively placed in Stage 2 because two separate lymph-node areas were involved. It was important to determine if lymph nodes and other organs under the diaphragm were also involved because this would put her in Stage 3. If she was in Stage 2, her treatment would be radiation only, but if she was in Stage 3 or 4 she would require chemotherapy.

Further tests (including a bone biopsy and a CAT scan, which is a very sensitive three-dimensional computer scan) convinced the oncologist that she was in Stage 3. Had any vital organ such as the lung, liver or bone marrow been involved, she would have been in Stage 4. Within a week after this patient was started on chemotherapy her neck mass disappeared; within two weeks her chest X ray was almost completely clear and within two months it was normal.

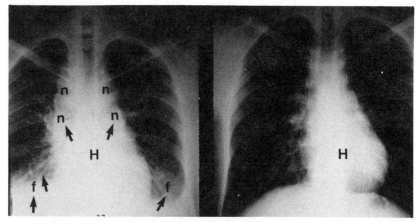

Response of Hodgkin's disease to chemotherapy. The white area (*H*) in the center of both X rays is the heart. In the X ray at left, light areas, *n* (cancerous lymph glands), and *f* (probably fluid in the lungs from Hodgkin's disease) surround the heart and make it appear bigger. These areas have completely cleared up in the X ray at right, taken just over five months later.

Another Hodgkin's disease patient was a twenty-six-year-old man who not only had a swelling that had progressed from his feet to his thigh but also had lumps about the size of small eggs in his neck, armpit and groin. X rays in July, 1977 showed very large tumors in his chest as well as tumors and fluid in one lung. His tumors responded very rapidly to chemotherapy consisting of MOPP, which he had for six months. All evidence of disease disappeared except for occasional night sweats, so he was switched to a different combination of medications known as ABVD for approximately six more months. The total length of his treatment was one year, and repeated re-examinations have shown the patient to have no symptoms and no trace of disease. The man was free of Hodgkin's disease in April, 1984 and is probably cured.

The availability of MOPP and ABVD signal a complete and dramatic change in the entire outlook for patients with Hodgkin's disease.

It can now be said with confidence that the cure rate of *cancer of the testicles* (testicular cancer), even at the moderately advanced stage, is approximately 80 percent. *All men with moderately early testicular cancer should be considered curable.* Even though tumors of the testicles comprise only about 1 percent of all malignancies in males, this cancer was a very serious problem until recently. It is estimated that 6,000 new cases were discovered in 1982 in the United States. This is the most common cancer in men between the ages of twenty-five and thirty-five and used to be the leading cause of cancer deaths of men in this age group. Consequently, the advances in conquering this disease are a tremendous achievement.

Cancer of the Testicles

Symptoms of the disease may not appear at all, or the patient may complain of a mass or heavy sensation in the testicles or, occasionally, pain in the testicles. It is not unusual for tumors of the testicles to resemble infections or inflammation and be treated as such. This inappropriate treatment may go on for months before the correct diagnosis is made.

Symptoms of Testicular Cancer

When testicular cancer is strongly suspected, diagnosis is made by the total removal of the testicle. A biopsy or partial removal of the testicle is not advisable because this would spread the tumor to the scrotum and the groin area. When a definite diagnosis is made, exploratory surgery may be necessary to examine the abdominal nodes. If the tumor was limited to the testicle, no further treatment is needed. *A patient who has had one testicle removed can have a normal sex life and can father children.* (Some of the body's organs—testicles and kidneys, for example—come in pairs, and if one is removed the other does the job quite efficiently by itself.)

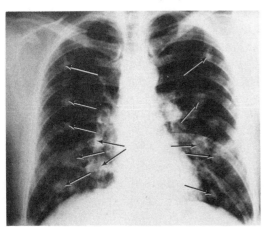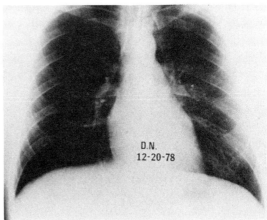

Response of testicular cancer to chemotherapy. Arrows in X ray at left show a number of white spots in the lungs. These spots, associated with testicular cancer, have completely disappeared in the X ray at right, taken after chemotherapy. (Courtesy of Kalish Kedia, M.D.)

Chemotherapy for Testicular Cancer   There are four main types of testicular cancer. The one called *seminoma* is particularly responsive to radiation—even when at an advanced stage. The other three types are not curable with local treatment alone (surgery) nor are they very responsive to radiation. However, with chemotherapy the survival rates improve, and Bleomycin and Vinblastine in combination seem to eradicate the disease in one third of the patients. By adding another drug, Cisplatinum, to the Bleomycin and Vinblastine, the percentage of success rises dramatically. Over 80 percent of the patients, even those with advanced testicular cancer that has metastasized to the lungs, show complete response. This treatment is now standardized, and in most cases can produce 80 to 100 percent response even if the tumor has already traveled to the lungs. (When testicular cancer metastasizes, it often goes to the lungs.)

74

As in the treatment of Hodgkin's disease, the medications used for treatment of this cancer can produce some very harsh side effects, particularly severe nausea and vomiting, which last approximately five hours. High fever and muscle aches may also be experienced, but precautions can be taken so that secondary side effects (such as transient kidney damage) are avoided. It is safe to say that in the hands of an experienced oncologist most of these side effects can easily be brought under control without any significant or permanent consequences.

A unique aspect of testicular cancer is that the tumor cells produce chemicals in the blood that can be tested to see whether, after treatment, there is still an active tumor or whether it has been completely eliminated. Consequently, the oncologist will know precisely when the treatment should be continued or discontinued with some margin of safety. These "marker" chemicals have helped improve the cure rate.

The few patients who relapse do so within the first year following treatment, and, in rare cases, after the first two years. Patients who have not shown any evidence of disease for two years after treatment has ended are probably completely cured. This devastating form of cancer, which attacks young men in the prime of life when they are economically productive and likely to be providing for small children, was a major killer throughout the mid-1970s but can now be classified as a curable disease.

The cure rate for *ovarian cancer* is extremely variable. Cures depend on how early the diagnosis is made, the aggressiveness of the disease and the appropriateness of the treatment. More than one out of every hundred women in the United States will eventually develop ovarian cancer, a percentage that may also be true in Canada. This cancer tends to occur in women over forty-five and is important because of the suffering and extremely high mortality rate associated with it. While it comprises only 25 percent of all gynecological cancers, it causes approximately 50 percent of all deaths due to these cancers. The principal reason for the high mortality rate is the delay in diagnosis.

The delay is usually due to the fact that patients do not experience any symptoms until late. Even if there are symptoms at an

Cancer of the Ovaries

early stage, they are vague: indigestion and abdominal discomfort. Neither the patient nor the primary physician may take these symptoms seriously. Furthermore, during the early stages of the disease, routine examinations and investigations may not give any clues to the problem. Consequently, these women often go to their family doctor complaining of mild abdominal pain and, after examinations that reveal nothing, are given antacids and tranquilizers. Even when the cancer is at the moderately advanced stage, routine examination may not show anything, which may also be true of more careful examination with several bowel X rays and internal examinations with an endoscope (a special instrument for this purpose). This may be true even when the patient has symptoms of nausea, vomiting and occasional diarrhea. Often it is only after the tumor can be easily felt or the patient has developed fluid in the abdomen that a correct diagnosis can be made. And even at this stage a cancer diagnosis may not be obvious on physical examination alone unless the patient is fairly thin (making it easy to feel the cancer) or the doctor happens to be particularly suspicious. Early diagnosis of ovarian cancer has been made easier in the past few years with the use of the intravenous pyelogram, which outlines the kidney and bladder; with CAT scans, which are computer scans of the abdomen and pelvis; and, especially, with ultrasound, which is a soundwave test for locating abnormal masses in the abdomen and pelvis.

High Cure Rate at an Early Stage

It is important to point out that ovarian cancer is one disease where teamwork is of utmost importance. The patient should seek help as soon as she has the slightest suspicion of any problem, and the family physician or internist should make every effort to arrive at a correct diagnosis. Early diagnosis is imperative in this disease since the cure rate is about 90 percent in Stage 1 (when the cancer is confined solely to the ovaries). Stage 2, where the tumor has spread beyond the ovaries to other organs in the pelvis but is still confined to the pelvic region, is also curable with the appropriate treatment. By Stage 3, the tumor has spread beyond the pelvis and gone into the abdominal cavity, and by Stage 4 the tumor has spread to some of the vital organs such as the lung, liver and bones. Until recently, the survival rate of women in Stage 3 was poor and in Stage 4 was nil. Seventy percent of the cases of this disease are generally not diagnosed until it has reached Stage 3 or 4.

The tremendous improvement in the treatment of ovarian cancers in recent years has resulted from better understanding of the growth and spread of the disease. In addition, progress has been made because of proper surgical treatment. The smaller the amount of tumor left behind after surgery, the better the chances for chemotherapy to succeed. Great successes have resulted from the use of combination chemotherapy and, particularly, from the development of newer drugs such as Cisplatinum and Hexamethylmelamine. Overall, the rate of response when Cisplatinum has been combined with two to four additional drugs is in excess of 70 to 80 percent during initial chemotherapy, if the tumor remaining after surgery is .78 inch or less in size. Chemotherapy is often so effective in some ovarian cancers that, even if the tumor is completely inoperable but the patient can be placed on drugs immediately after a biopsy, the tumor size may shrink significantly and surgery can subsequently be performed to completely remove all of the visible tumor.

The side effects of the chemotherapy depend on the particular combination of drugs. These side effects usually include nausea and vomiting, hair loss, numbness and tingling in the fingers and toes. Patients should have a lot of fluids to avoid dehydration and kidney damage if Cisplatinum is used.

In November, 1976, I saw a fifty-one-year-old woman for cancer of the ovary. Six months prior to the diagnosis, she had had her yearly examination and Pap test, which appeared to be normal. Two weeks before her admission she noted a pelvic mass. Her X rays were normal except for an area that indicated some pressure on the bladder due to displacement by what we now suspected was a pelvic tumor. During surgery, which took place almost immediately, a 14-inch tumor was found, which burst during the operation, spilling the tumor into the abdomen (not an unusual occurrence). The patient underwent chemotherapy with large doses of Cytoxan once a month for a year. Toward the end of the treatment she developed severe nausea and vomiting, requiring overnight hospital admission for dehydration and intramuscular anti-nausea medication, but, at the completion of the treatment, all examinations including a second-look operation revealed no evidence of tumor. This woman is probably cured. More important, medications are available that would most likely produce complete response if this tumor ever came back.

The outcome of the treatment of the patient in the next case illustrates a point about cancer treatment that I cannot overemphasize—no one should ever give up hope prematurely if there is the slightest chance of controlling the disease.

Success Despite Complicating Factors

This is the case of a woman who, in the spring of 1976, was found not only to have moderately advanced cancer of the ovary (Stage 3) but also to have had severe damage from a heart attack. Both the cancer and the heart condition were successfully treated at that time and in 1982 the patient was in excellent health without any cancer symptoms whatsoever.

On May 10, 1976, she was admitted to the hospital for pain and a mass in the right lower abdomen. A diagnosis of appendicitis was made. During the operation, both ovaries were found to have cancer that had already spread from the ovaries to the abdomen. At the same time it was discovered that she had had a "silent"—unknown—heart attack. After recovering from surgery, the woman was started on chemotherapy. Three months later she had progressively severe heart failure, anemia and fluid in her lungs. She was sent to a heart specialist because the heart problem was not responding to the usual treatment. The following November she underwent open-heart surgery that also involved removal of a large blood clot and dead heart tissue (an aneurysm). The patient did exceedingly well after the operation and continued with chemotherapy for one year.

In 1978 she moved to Arizona but came back to visit in June, 1981. She reported to her oncologist that she had been traveling all over the country with her husband while also participating in many programs in her community. She looked absolutely terrific and stated that she had no problems whatsoever and, as of July, 1983 (the last time I heard from her), she was still in excellent health. If, because of her advanced cancer combined with a serious heart problem, she or her doctors had vetoed aggressive treatment, she would have died a long time ago.

In the past, a diagnosis of advanced ovarian cancer signified certain death preceded by a considerable amount of suffering. Now,

78

with aggressive treatment, many women, even with this cancer in advanced stages, can lead very productive and normal or near-normal lives for years.

The cure rate of *breast cancer* depends very much on the stage *Breast Cancer* of the disease when it is discovered. The five-year survival rate is nearly 85 percent if the tumor is limited to the breast, about 60 percent if the lymph nodes are involved, and 10 percent if distant metastasis has taken place by the time of diagnosis. About 50 percent of newly diagnosed patients have local disease, 40 percent have lymph-node (or regional) involvement, and 10 percent have advanced disease. These survival-rate figures are from 1960 to 1971, but they still underscore the need for early diagnosis and proper treatment of breast cancer.

In the U.S. there are about 100,000 new cases of breast cancer each year. Although this cancer can attack any age group, it concentrates particularly on women from ages forty to forty-five, and is the leading cause of death in women in that age bracket. Until the 1970s there was no great improvement in the long-term survival rate of breast-cancer patients, a sad situation that was due to a lack of understanding of the biology of this kind of cancer. Breast cancer tends to spread early, but *after* it becomes detectable.

Once breast cancer has spread outside the breast tissue itself (for example, into the adjacent lymph nodes) there is a great likelihood that it has also spread far beyond the lymph nodes. This is why radical surgery (removal of the breast, surrounding muscles and nearby lymph nodes) and extensive local radiation to the breast area after surgery have not improved the survival rate of patients who already showed signs of metastasis at the time of initial treatment. This knowledge, along with new strategy in breast cancer treatment, has greatly improved chances of survival.

The most common symptom of breast cancer is a lump *Symptoms* discovered either by the patient or her physician. A newly discovered lump in a woman under twenty-five years of age is likely to be benign; in a patient sixty-five or older it is very likely to be malignant. A lump in the armpit may be a sign of advanced disease.

With or without a lump, any breast pain that is not usually associated with the woman's menses may be another sign. Retraction, dimpling or an inward pulling of the skin or nipple is a clear warning. Other signs of breast cancer may be itching, cracking or soreness of the nipple. In rare cases called inflammatory breast cancer, there may be no distinct lump, but part of the breast may appear to be hot, red and firm, which may suggest an infection—but treatment for an infection will not be successful if the problem is cancer.

Regardless of the patient's age, if a new lump or mass is discovered, it should be thoroughly investigated. There are several ways of dealing with a breast lump. In the first place, in most cases the lump will turn out to be benign or just a cyst. If benign fluid is removed from a cyst, and the fluid does not reaccumulate, no further treatment is needed except for observation. A needle biopsy to remove some fluid can be done under local anesthesia in a doctor's office. If tumor cells appear in the needle biopsy, or if the lump is not clearly a cyst, a mammogram is done. A mammogram is a special X ray of the breast that can pick up early cancer and can also distinguish benign from malignant breast masses. There is, however, a small chance of missing breast cancer on a mammogram. Therefore a breast mass or a suspicious area that has the usual features of malignancy should be fully investigated. Sometimes a biopsy should be performed in spite of negative mammogram because other factors indicate the need for further investigation.

Conference
Before Surgery
Prior to further investigation, a pre-surgical conference should be next in order for the doctor to explain all the treatment options, including treatment after surgery if cancer is suspected. This pre-surgical conference is very important in order to minimize the shock and anguish associated with breast removal. It used to be common for a woman to go into surgery hoping and expecting only a biopsy and waking up to find a breast missing. We now know enough about breast cancer treatment to discuss and advise patients about various options.

If a lump turns out to have been cancerous, and there is a spread to the lymph nodes or beyond, the patient will be advised to undergo chemotherapy. Patients who receive chemotherapy early, when the disease is present only in microscopic amounts, not only stay free of cancer longer but also live longer. Chemotherapy has also improved the condition of patients with more advanced breast cancer. Combining three or four different medications simultaneously has increased the response rate to 60 to 80 percent. While chemotherapy does not produce a significant number of cures, in very advanced breast cancer it can improve the quality of life for many thousands of women if they are in the hands of qualified specialists.

One valuable advance in the treatment of breast cancer in the past few years has been the pinpointing of breast tumors whose growth is stimulated by female hormones. Now it is not only possible to take chemotherapeutic drugs that neutralize the effect of the hormones, but the drugs are easy to take—in tablet form. These drugs prevent the hormones from providing nourishment to the breast cancer cells (see final section of Chapter 4 on anti-estrogen treatment).

Success in Spite of Bone and Liver Metastasis

Many patients think that when the tumor has traveled to the bones or the liver this means the end is near. The following case shows that this is not necessarily true.

A forty-six-year-old woman had a mastectomy in January, 1975. The tumor had metastasized to only one of twenty lymph nodes. The patient received radiation treatments, and a bone scan taken a year later was negative, showing no sign of cancer. However, in December, 1977 the patient developed some bone pain, and bone and liver scans showed considerable metastasis to the spine, ribs and liver. After a two-hour discussion, she and her husband were finally convinced that she could be helped and that her condition was not completely hopeless, as they had originally believed. She began chemotherapy, responded, and, as she continued, was prescribed anti-estrogens to add to the treatment. After two years all evidence of cancer disappeared both from the bone and the liver, and she continued to be without any detectable tumor six and a half years later, in April, 1984.

This is a good example of how patients may do very well even though there is extensive cancer throughout the body. It is also important to point out that following surgery, this patient had only one out of twenty lymph nodes involved; yet, after two years, she had extensive tumors all over her body. The fact that she responded so well to chemotherapy suggests that she might have been much better off if she had been treated with chemotherapy soon after her initial surgery. Neither the patient nor the family doctor is to blame for not starting chemotherapy early; all this means is that there have been drastic changes in the treatment of breast cancer over the past several years.

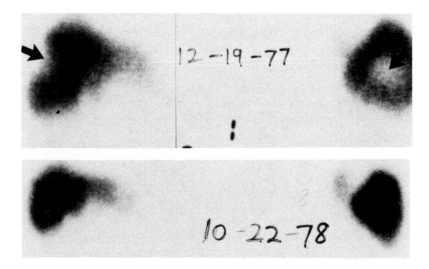

Response to chemotherapy of a breast cancer that had spread to the liver. Each photo shows front and side views of a liver scan. The white area in the center of the scan at the top right (arrow) is a large tumor. (As an indication of its size, the average liver is bigger than the head of a six-year-old child.) In the bottom scan, taken ten months later, the white area has disappeared and the scan shows a normal liver.

I should caution that this case of bone and liver metastasis completely clearing up is an exception and not the rule. But clearly "miracles" can be accomplished only if the patient begins the treatment and does not despair. Chemotherapy has improved the cure rate of tumors that have spread to the lymph nodes and has also reduced the need for radical surgery that was quite common in the past.

Lung Cancer   *Lung cancer* is one of the most serious forms of cancer in the western hemisphere simply because of the large numbers of people it afflicts and the high mortality rate of those who develop it. In the U.S. alone, about 140,000 new cases are diagnosed each year. The major cause is cigarette smoking, and the age at which the cancer shows up can be as low as thirty. There are four types of lung cancer: *small-cell cancer, squamous-cell cancer, adenocarcinoma* and *large-cell cancer.*

Symptoms of lung cancer may be a dry cough, bloody sputum, chest pain, shortness of breath or recurrent pneumonia that does not clear up even with proper antibiotic treatment. Often symptoms due to metastasis such as bone pain or headaches may occur.

Diagnosis can be made on a chest X ray followed by a lung biopsy. Sometimes a bone-marrow biopsy will be done in order to determine the cell type.

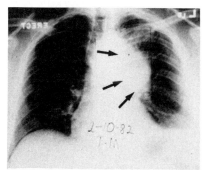 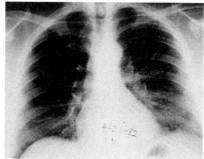

Response of a small-cell lung cancer to chemotherapy. The white mass indicated by arrows in the X ray at left (a tumor) has disappeared in the X ray at right, taken two months later. This patient received a very high dose of Methotrexate and CCNU in combination with other chemotherapeutic drugs.

Small-cell Cancer

Of the four types of lung cancer, approximately 25 percent are small-cell cancer, so named because of the size of the cancer cells. About 25,000 new cases are diagnosed in the United States every year. This is the lung cancer that is the most responsive to chemotherapy. Aggressive use of combination chemotherapy has resulted in 25 percent of the patients with early metastasis surviving for two years. Even though the percentage of cure is by no means as high as with other cancers, the significant fact is the improvement in the quality of life for these patients.

Death occurs because small-cell cancer grows extremely fast and can double in size in four weeks. Until the last few years, the disease was inevitably fatal not only because of the rapid growth of the cells but also because they tended to metastasize to other parts of the body early in the course of the disease. Death could occur as early as eight weeks or less from the time of diagnosis if the cancer was left untreated or if treatment was not effective. Surgery or radiation alone were not very helpful, even at the early stages, because they tended to be only localized. Treatment of small-cell cancer between 1931 to 1971 at the renowned Sloan-Kettering Memorial Hospital in New York revealed that for 93 percent of these patients, operations would be useless. Of the remaining 7 percent that were operated on, only two patients survived five years in the entire forty-year period. However, in the late 1970s the dismal outlook began to change. The use of combination chemotherapy with such drugs as Cytoxan, CCNU, Methotrexate, Oncovin, Adriamycin and VePeside (etoposide) has produced dramatic results in many patients. When careful radiation is added to this combination chemotherapy in selected patients, the results are even more encouraging: a response of about 75 to 90 percent in patients whose cancer is limited to one lung. Unfortunately, the disease returns to most of the patients who show a good initial response. At present only about 25 percent of the patients who have small-cell lung cancer limited to one lung, and who show complete response, remain free of disease for over two years. Some of these are probably cured.

The side effects of combination chemotherapy include a severely low blood count as well as whatever other side effects those particular drugs would have.

Hopeful Future for Former Smoker   One success story concerning small-cell lung cancer involves a woman who had smoked about two packs of cigarettes a day for more than twenty years. In October, 1981, at age fifty-eight, she had a lump in her neck that had grown to the size of an egg in about five weeks. She also had a spot about the size of a nickel in her chest. She had no other symptoms, and a test for distant metastasis indicated no further spread. She was placed on large doses of chemotherapy administered in two parts to minimize side effects. Six weeks later, the tumors in the neck and chest had disappeared completely. Her chances for long-term remission are excellent. As of this writing, almost three years later, she is free of the disease.

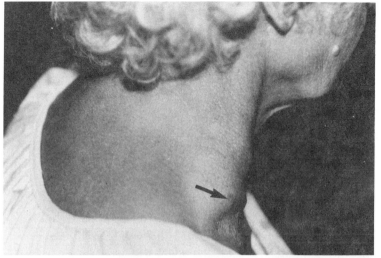

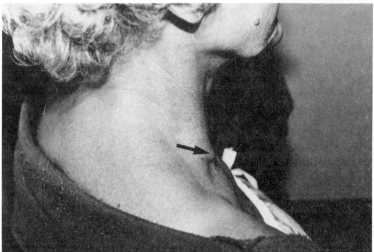

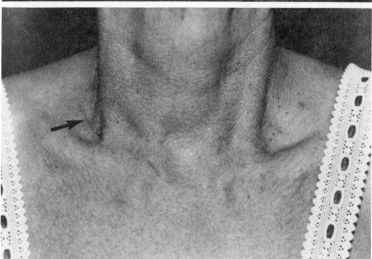

A particularly dramatic example of the effectiveness of chemotherapy in a case of small-cell cancer that had spread to the lymph nodes of the neck. The large lump indicated by the arrow in the top photo (taken in October, 1981) had shrunk considerably just two and a half weeks later (center) and completely disappeared by the following December. Only a scar remains.

Even though the cure rate for small-cell lung cancer is relatively low, it does respond to chemotherapy. It is only a matter of time before different types of medication used in the right combination will begin to produce a greater percentage of cures, and it is highly likely that within the near future the majority of patients with small-cell cancer (and whose disease is detected at a reasonably early stage) will enjoy a higher rate of cure.

Squamous-cell Lung Cancer and Adenocarcinoma

The other types of lung cancer, squamous-cell cancer and adenocarcinoma, are not as responsive to treatment in the advanced stage as small-cell cancer. Squamous-cell cancer (*squamous* comes from the Latin and means "scaly") tends not to grow as fast as small-cell cancer, and the few cases that are discovered early, before metastasis, can be cured with surgery. Radiation treatment is often effective in giving relief from symptoms. Until the 1980s, chemotherapy was not used much in the treatment of either squamous-cell cancer or adenocarcinoma. Now, though, doctors are frequently seeing good to excellent responses when chemotherapy is used to treat squamous-cell cancer and occasional dramatic responses when used for adenocarcinoma. However, many of these responses are not long-lasting and cannot be translated into cures. Combination chemotherapy using Cisplatinum as the principal drug has produced some encouraging results in selected patients who are well enough to tolerate rigorous chemotherapy.

The challenge now is to find new and more powerful medications to include in the combination in order to get more responses and to improve the chances of cures. In addition, ways of improving the body's immune system could prevent the return of the cancer and could prevent relapses in patients who have had excellent initial responses. (See the sections on interferon and monoclonal antibodies toward the end of Chapter 9.)

Success Stories

Examples of what aggressive treatment can achieve are two of my patients with lung cancer, one with squamous-cell cancer, one with adenocarcinoma, who both responded well to chemotherapy.

The first is a sixty-seven-year-old man who was advised, when diagnosed in 1980 with squamous-cell lung cancer, to undergo chemotherapy because of evidence of metastasis. The man refused treatment and sought no further medical attention. Three years later his wife came to me with painful breast cancer that had metastasized to the bone. She was given mild oral chemotherapy, to which she responded very well, and the pain disappeared. At this point the husband decided to see what could be done for him. He now had chest pain and bone metastasis. He was put on chemotherapy and has shown an excellent initial response—the tumor is almost completely cleared up. His symptoms have totally disappeared and he is leading a normal life, as if he had never heard of cancer.

The second case is a sixty-year-old woman whose adenocarcinoma had metastasized to the liver. In October, 1982 she was started on combination chemotherapy; within weeks the severe pain she had been suffering, and which required heavy doses of narcotics, comcompletely subsided. By April, 1983 she appeared to be clear of all visible tumors. Localized radiation was given to the lung and liver to destroy any remaining tumors. The patient tolerated both the chemotherapy and radiation exceedingly well, only once experiencing nausea and vomiting from the chemotherapy and on one occasion having a severe sore throat and prolonged fatigue. When a new tumor appeared in another part of the lung in September, 1983, she was returned to chemotherapy and as of this writing in July, 1984, she is stable, with a good partial remission, and leading an active, productive life, although she takes a bit longer to recover from chemotherapy. In the winter of '84 she drove from Cleveland to Florida and drove an additional thousand miles within Florida. Right now she still manages one of the largest dance studios in Ohio.

The plan for the future treatment of this patient is to take some of her bone marrow and store it. She will be given a megadose of chemotherapy in the hope of producing a lasting response; in order to prevent an extremely low blood count from the megadose, she will be given back her own bone marrow. Because she has responded so well to chemotherapy in the past, it is very likely she will respond well to the megadose.

Another form of lung cancer—specifically, *cancer of the lung lining*—is *mesothelioma*. This cancer, which is strongly linked to asbestos exposure, is difficult to treat, but doctors are now beginning to see an occasional excellent response when Cisplatinum and

Mesothelioma

Adriamycin are used as the principal drugs in combination chemotherapy. A case that comes to mind is a sixty-three-year-old woman
who was found to have mesothelioma in September, 1983, and
started combination chemotherapy. She appeared to have an unusual sensitivity to Cisplatinum, so extra precautions were taken to
minimize the side effects. The Cisplatinum was discontinued in January, 1984, with milder chemotherapy on a monthly basis still going
on as of July, 1984. This patient was able to go to her winter home
and is tolerating her treatment quite well.

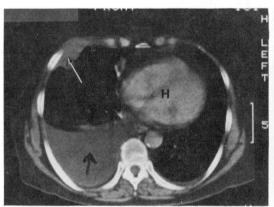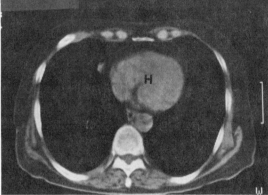

Mesothelioma (cancer of the lung lining) cleared up by chemotherapy. These
two CAT scans show a cross-section of the upper chest area, with the heart labelled *H*. The light gray areas indicated by arrows (left) are cancerous tumors
and fluid—gone four months later (right).

*Colon and Rectal
Cancers*   When the medical statistics for 1984 have been collected, they
probably will show that 120,000 to 130,000 cases of colon or rectal
cancer occurred in the United States in that year, making these among
the most common kinds of cancer.

These cancers (commonly grouped together as colorectal
cancers) have been receiving a lot of recent attention because
authorities suspect there may be a direct connection between these
two cancers and diet. Thorough analysis seems to suggest that groups
of people whose diets are high in fat and low in fiber—
for example, the populations of Canada, the U.S., the United Kingdom
and other Western countries—are much more likely to have colorectal cancers than groups of people whose diets are low in fat and high in
fiber. It is possible that a low-fiber-high-fat diet may change the

88

bacterial climate of the gut, allowing production of cancer-causing elements in the bowel. Some members of the medical community are beginning to recommend that patients decrease the amounts of fats in their diets while increasing the amounts of whole grains, fruits, and raw vegetables.

Whatever its cause, colorectal cancer, with certain exceptions, is rare in people under forty. One exception is people who have inherited a tendency to these two cancers; studies show that one out of five colorectal cancer patients comes from a family in which a close relative has had the disease. The only other person under forty who might develop the disease would be someone who has had ulcerative colitis, numerous polyps, or certain apparently benign colon tumors.

The early warning signs of colorectal cancer, which are usually *Symptoms* easy to recognize, are all too often blamed on hemorrhoids or are simply ignored until the symptoms become painful. Symptoms include bright red rectal bleeding, changes in bowel habits such as constipation or diarrhea, rectal pain, a feeling of incomplete evacuation of the stools, or severe abdominal cramps that are partially relieved by bowel movements.

In general, these last two symptoms (which are signs of bowel blockage), along with bright red bleeding, tend to be symptoms of cancer on the left side of the colon. Because the right side of the colon, which is for storage, is more expandable, patients with cancer on that side may experience no symptoms until the tumor is in an advanced stage and has metastasized. Once in a while a tumor on the right side will be large enough that the doctor or patient will notice a lump, and occasionally, if it is very bulky, it will cause bowel blockage. Eighty percent of all colorectal cancer patients will at some time experience bleeding of the colon and rectum (gastrointestinal bleeding), which results in unusually dark stools due to old blood and may lead to progressive weakness and anemia.

Early warning signs, because they do not seem dramatic, are easy to overlook. Cases might be a man over forty who always had one bowel movement a day and now has one, without any discomfort, only every third or fourth day. Or a woman of sixty who has had normal bowel movements and never been bothered by diarrhea but now has new bowel habits with occasional diarrhea for a month or more. Or a normally vigorous housewife who now gets tired and can hardly complete her day's chores. Such people should not blame these changes on stress, age or, if they have rectal bleeding, on hemorrhoids. These signs should be checked out. Three fourths of all colorectal cancer deaths could probably be prevented by early diagnosis and proper treatment.

The diagnosis of colorectal cancer is usually quite straightforward and may be done by a rectal examination, examination with a flexible tube, or radiographic examination involving a barium enema or a tube. Occasionally it is simply a matter of the patient or doctor finding a mass on the right side.

Treatment: Surgery   Surgery, which is the only sure method of cure for colorectal cancer, is very effective if the tumor is caught at an early stage and treated promptly. One method of determining how far a tumor has advanced is known as Dukes staging. Dukes stage A means the cancer is confined to the wall of the colon or rectum. A cancer found at this stage will have a cure rate of 75 to 100 percent. Dukes stage B means the cancer has grown through the inner wall of the colon and reached the outside wall, but has not gone into the lymph glands. This stage has a 50 to 70 percent possibility of five-year survival. Dukes C means metastasis into the nearby or regional lymph nodes, and the five-year survival rate becomes about 25 percent. However, another factor is involved: the degree of malignancy. If the degree of malignancy is low, the five-year survival rate is about 80 percent; if intermediate, 60 percent; high, 25 percent.

When colorectal cancer is treated surgically, the diseased section of the colon is removed, and the remaining colon sewed together. Occasionally the cancer is located in the lower part of the rectum where there is nothing left to sew together after surgery. Such a situation requires a *colostomy*, a surgically made colon opening in the abdominal wall for elimination of the stools. As surgical techniques improve, there is less and less need for colostomies. Colostomy patients will find that nearly all hospitals have at least one nurse trained in the care of colostomy who is always available, and the American Cancer Society has a good program for the education and emotional support of such patients.

The main reason for radiation in the treatment of colorectal cancer is prevention of, or treatment of, local metastasis. The usefulness of radiation in colorectal cancer is limited to the rectum and the lower part of the sigmoid colon (which is the part of the colon just above the rectum). In these two areas, there is less chance of radiation damaging the sensitive small bowels. Half of the deaths from sigmoid or rectal cancer are due to problems of the cancer returning or growing in these locations, so careful radiation for patients with early metastasis will not only ease discomfort but will help reverse these statistics.

Radiation and Chemotherapy

The chemotherapy available today is not very effective in the treatment of colorectal cancer. The drug that has been principally used since the mid-1960s has been 5FU. Several combinations of drugs have also been tried, but they have not been any more effective than 5FU, and I hope that we will soon see more imaginative use of current medications as well as new drugs.

With individualized treatment, even advanced cases can respond well. See Chapter 3, page 20, for the case history of a man whose unusually large tumor of the colon was treated with surgery, radiation, and chemotherapy—and who, as the photograph shows, is leading a productive life with significant remission.

Individualized Treatment Pays Off

As far as colorectal cancer is concerned, the major effort of the medical world at this point should be directed toward early discovery of the tumor and complete curative surgical removal of it. Since three quarters of colorectal cancers give early warning symptoms, and since two thirds of colorectal cancers can be easily felt during an examination, it is reasonable to hope that oncologists encountering colorectal cancers will find them still in the earliest stage.

Since it's impossible to discuss every kind of cancer, I will end this chapter with a a point that cannot be stated too often: *Each case of cancer must be looked at as unique.* By being alert to those patients who might beat the odds by responding to special or aggressive treatment, medical teams can occasionally produce amazing responses with cancers that would not usually be sensitive to treatment. On the other hand, patients who are obviously not going to

Every Case Is Different

respond should be treated with the goal of being kept as comfortable as possible.

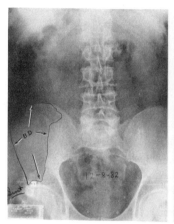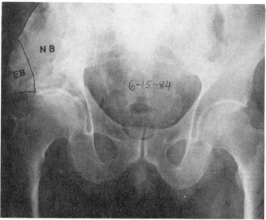

Response of multiple myeloma (bone cancer) to treatment. In the X ray at left, taken in December, 1982, every bone is extensively involved with cancer, and two-thirds of the right hip have been completely destroyed (*BD*). The X ray at right shows marked healing, with new bone formation (*NB*) along with extra bone formation (*EB*) after radiation and chemotherapy.

Note: In lung X rays, light areas indicate cancerous tissue; dark areas, healthy tissues. In bone X rays, however, the opposite holds: dark areas are cancerous, and light areas show healthy bone. The reason for this seeming contradiction is that X rays show areas of contrasting density, and a lung tumor has more density than healthy lung tissue, whereas healthy bone is denser than cancerous bone.

Successes with Pancreatic Cancer and Bone Cancer

In my own experience, two cases of beating the odds immediately come to mind. The first is a seventy-three-year-old woman with cancer of the pancreas that was found to consist mainly of a type of cancer cell not usually found in this cancer.* I felt that the patient, after her surgery, could tolerate the chemotherapeutic drug that has been effective against these particular cells in other kinds of cancer. When the chemotherapy ended, she was given radiation to eliminate what showed up on a CAT scan as a possible remaining bit of tumor. Now, two and a half years later, she appears to have no sign that the tumor has returned.

The second example is a man with bone cancer (multiple

*As a matter of medical record, this was predominantly a squamous-cell type of adeno-squamous cancer with adjacent-node metastisis. The diagnosis was made at a teaching hospital.

myeloma), whose entire skeletal system had been attacked by the cancer and whose right hip had been extensively damaged. He has been treated with radiation sandwiched in between chemotherapy treatments. He has done exceedingly well and is without symptoms.

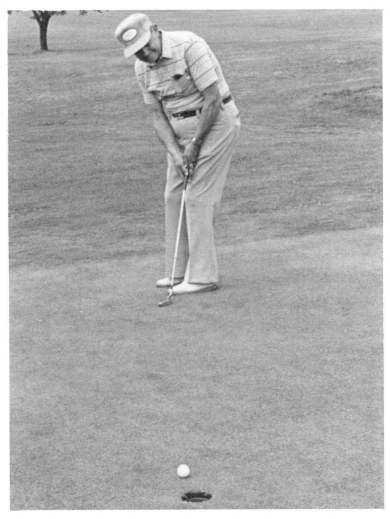

This is the man whose X rays are the preceding pair — a man who now no longer even needs a cane. When asked if he would be willing to be photographed for this book, he said, "I'd be delighted to have my picture used to give hope to other patients."

These two case histories show that even patients with advanced cancer for which there is no certain cure can enjoy long-term remission with excellent quality of life. The fact that such patients respond to chemotherapy is the first step toward finding a cure for these difficult tumors. I hope that the next few years will bring new treatment methods, more potent chemicals, and ways of getting the human body to wipe out the cancer cells that remain in the system after initial excellent responses to chemotherapy.

CHAPTER EIGHT

Living with Cancer and Chemotherapy

The lifestyle of a cancer patient depends on several factors including the type of cancer, the availability of effective treatment, the duration of remission and, most importantly, the patient's mental outlook. Cancer should be accepted as a chronic disease—it is not a punishment. The initial anger, frustration, self-pity and "Why me?" reactions are understandable and normal. But there is no justification for the sense of guilt or shame that some people feel. After all, with cancer as with most chronic diseases, for the most part no one has any control over who gets it. Most cancer patients are able to carry on with normal activities and with as little disruption as can be managed. A positive attitude toward life and an ability to take each day as it comes can make the difference between enjoying life's pleasures and dreading each sunrise.

The expense of treating cancer can be enormous. A major expense is the hidden costs due to loss of a job because of prejudice and discrimination or because of disability or absence from work due to the illness and the treatment. A more direct burden may be due to inadequate or nonexistent medical insurance.

Financial Considerations

The cost of a typical hospital outpatient treatment for breast or lymph cancer with several drugs varies from $60 to over $300 for each visit, and several visits may be required each month. This cost is high partly because of the drug costs to the provider; for example, a 15-unit (or 15-milligram) vial of Bleomycin is $65, a 50-milligram vial of Adriamycin is $85 and Mitomycin (only a 20-milligram vial) is $165. Besides these costs are those for X rays and blood tests, which are absolutely essential for following the progress of a patient undergoing treatment. All totaled, the costs for the treatment of cancer may become a serious financial burden for patients with or without medical insurance. The primary means for paying these bills is, of course, insurance. Ideally, everyone should find out the extent and limitations of their medical coverage before any illness occurs. The fact that a patient has insurance means very little if it is only a bare-bones policy or one that pays little of the cost of the appropriate treatment. Most cancer patients do have adequate coverage so that they have no, or only nominal, out-of-pocket expenses.

Importance of Knowing Insurance Coverage

No one wants to be in the position of a newly married twenty-six-year-old man I know of who was diagnosed as having a particularly aggressive type of lymph-system cancer. His insurance was found to be very inadequate. It stipulated (in fine print) that it would pay only $600 for surgical fees for a single disease over a six-month period. This young man's two initial surgeries for diagnosis and treatment cost over $1,200. The policy also classified chemotherapy as surgery, so he had no coverage at all for his chemotherapy during the first six months after surgery. Neither the patient nor his insurance agent was aware of this problem until the chemotherapy was administered in the hospital. It therefore bears repeating that everyone should become familiar with the scope of coverage in any health-insurance policy.

In addition to the extent of coverage, a patient should note the limitations. Some policies exclude coverage for outpatient chemotherapy. If a policy states that it includes "major medical" expenses then, usually, practically all outpatient expenses will be paid up to 80 percent of reasonable charges. This would include office visits, drugs, prosthetic devices (artificial parts of the body) and so on. A patient who has this major medical coverage would have relatively little to pay out of pocket. This amount would be the 20 percent and the usual $100 to $250 per person or $200 to $500 per family deductible per year.

Some policies restrict treatment to a specific hospital. These types of policies are generally tied to HMOs (health maintenance organizations). The advantage of an HMO is that the physicians who work at the designated hospital are salaried, and no additional costs are required for the physicians' services. However, a patient may want to be treated by a specialist who does not work at the stated hospital; in such cases where the patient selects an outside physician, this cost would not be covered by the insurance unless the patient were referred by the HMO.

Any problem concerning hospital bills should be explained to the health-care provider, especially the hospital, before treatment is started, in order to avoid any surprises. Every hospital has a social service department and staff to help the patient get access to resources provided by the hospital or the community. For example, the young man with lymph-system cancer was allowed to get necessary medications from the hospital pharmacy at cost, and the oncologist provided the complicated treatments in his office on an outpatient basis, thus considerably reducing the unfortunate man's expenses. The oncologist provided these services free until the patient's new insurance became effective four months later. In another case, a woman preferred to have major cancer surgery done at a community hospital that did not participate in her insurance company's HMO plan. The hospital providing the surgery arranged for her to pay $170 a month for a year. All other hospital expenses above this monthly payment were waived for that year—over $10,000. Her oncologist also charged only a nominal fee for her services until new insurance went into effect. Such assistance, of course, was based strictly on the individual patients' needs, which were particularly severe in these two cases.

Discussing Financial Problems in Advance

Either hospital staff or an attending physician can direct a patient toward community-service organizations such as the American Cancer Society, which is a great source of help since it can pay for all cancer-related medication (except chemotherapy) up to about $50 a

Outside Financial Help

97

month. Such organizations may also provide necessary equipment such as hospital beds and prosthetic devices as well as social assistance through home help programs. Specific associations such as the Leukemia Society also provide similar assistance but often, to qualify for help, the patient must have a disease of major interest to that particular organization. As a rule, a patient can receive excellent care at "teaching hospitals"—those associated with major medical colleges and universities. At some teaching hospitals many types of treatment are given at very nominal costs, depending upon the patient's financial condition and the research taking place there.

A patient should always explain any financial difficulty to the attending physician. If possible, some physicians will make special individual payment arrangements or will suspend payment for a patient in dire need of their services until problems of inadequate insurance are solved. Others will accept the 80 percent insurance payment without requiring the other 20 percent in cases where coverage is only 80 percent and real financial difficulty exists. If medications are not too expensive, drug-manufacturing companies will *occasionally* provide free samples for a physician to use for a specific patient who needs financial help.

A patient should never hesitate to discuss financial matters with his or her oncologist; after all, a physician is concerned not only with the physical health of the patient and the patient's family but also with their emotional and financial well-being. Finding ways to reduce or eliminate depression and discouragement due to money matters can be a major factor in successful treatment.

Employment   I suspect that the general public is unaware of how often during, say, the course of a month's business, they come into contact with people who are being, or recently were, treated for cancer. Cancer does not mean the end of the patient's work life, and in many cases does not even mean interruption.

Of my own patients who have needed surgery, a substantial number of those who worked prior to their illness were able to return to work in a month after the surgery or diagnosis. With few exceptions, I encourage patients to continue working as long as they are physically able. In fact, most cancer patients are able to do anything they were doing before they became ill. Whenever possible, I schedule patients for treatment in such a way that they lose as little time from work as possible. Usually it's not difficult to accommodate patients who are employed and do not want to take much time off for their treatments. Many patients are able to have their treatment in the office early in the day before they go to work or later in the afternoon after leaving work. Of course, this type of schedule depends to some extent on the medications being taken and how well the patient can handle any side effects.

One admirable woman who lost her husband to cancer many years ago found at the age of fifty that she herself had developed breast cancer. For the four years that she was taking intermittent chemotherapy, she would begin her treatment days by coming to my office at about eight o'clock in the morning, getting her treatment and then driving sixty miles to work. She had been in remission for about one and a half years when the cancer returned. This time she required a more potent medication, which resulted in complete loss of her hair, and later on she required a full course of radiation therapy. This woman is now in complete remission and has not needed chemotherapy for some time. It is significant that throughout the entire treatment, she carried on with normal days of full-time employment. She was so successful that not even her immediate supervisor was aware that she was undergoing cancer treatment. The patient was the only female executive in her company and did not want people feeling sorry for her or treating her differently because she was undergoing treatment for cancer. In addition to working full time, she is an excellent artist and even when on chemotherapy did a lot of paintings in her spare time. Most of these she gave to friends, including three excellent paintings for her oncologist. "I'm not going to sit down feeling sorry for myself. I'll continue to be busy and help other people," she said.

Most of the patients I see are able to carry on with this type of normal activity because they have a very determined, healthy and positive attitude toward their situation.

A Case of Not Allowing Treatment to Interrupt Work

Cancer is not simply a personal burden—rather it is a matter involving family and friends. It is very important that relatives and

Personal Relationships

friends realize that cancer is *not* contagious and as far as anyone knows, does not spread to others. No one is going to catch cancer from another person, so there is no need for relatives and friends to abandon the patient because he or she has cancer. Not only is there a need for kindness and understanding to be shown to the patient; in turn, it is equally important for the patient to be cooperative and helpful to family and friends. By far the largest percentage of family members and close friends do their very best to assist the patient. A few words of appreciation expressed by all concerned can go a long way in helping everyone cope with the situation.

I think I speak for most oncologists when I strongly urge patients to be honest with family members and close friends. Attempting to hide the truth or cover up feelings of anxiety simply does more harm than good, despite intentions for the best. Patients who freely discuss their problems with those they trust seem to be better able to face the physical and emotional aspects of cancer.

Need for Open Communication

In December, 1981, I had a patient who was tolerating chemotherapy very poorly—not only was she confined to her home but she was sick for ten days following each treatment. In addition, her husband complained of abdominal cramps and diarrhea. Both of them were upset and particularly anxious one day when they came in for an appointment. An hour of discussion with the two of them gradually revealed the fact that they were not communicating with each other about her illness. She had been diagnosed as having cancer that involved the liver and bone, and she stated in tears that her previous oncologist had told her that she only had two years to live. A year had already gone by, so this was her final year. She had been making every effort to conceal her feelings and this information from her children, sisters, parents and husband. It was apparent that her state of mind was not only an obstacle to chemotherapy but was a source of hidden anxiety for her husband, who was also reacting physically. After being assured that her condition was not that grim and that, in fact, her cancer was responding very favorably to the treatment, she became a completely different person. Her more positive outlook on life greatly improved her relationship with her family, and her husband's physical problems subsided—as did her severe reaction to chemotherapy. A patient's attitudes will inevitably affect the entire family as well as the patient.

Sexual relationships should not be given up simply because a partner has developed cancer. As mentioned earlier, cancer is not contagious and normal sexual activity certainly will not spread it. Sometimes the disease itself or the chemotherapy may decrease the sexual drive but this effect is often temporary, especially among patients who are responding well to treatment. An oncologist will advise a patient when sexual relationships are inadvisable and for how long. Do not hesitate to discuss the matter with your doctor.

All women who are in their reproductive years should take precautions against pregnancy while receiving chemotherapy. Chemotherapy, remember, interferes with rapidly dividing cells. A fetus grows by rapid cell division, so some chemotherapeutic drugs can cause damage to a developing fetus or even lead to spontaneous abortion. I should add that I know of many apparently normal children born to mothers who had leukemia and were receiving chemotherapy; nevertheless, since the long-term effect of these drugs on children is unknown, caution seems to be the best course of action at this time.

The patient who is well nourished tolerates cancer treatment much better than the one who is weak and eating poorly. Clearly, patients should be encouraged to eat as much wholesome food as they can get and to eat what agrees with them. Pamphlets about nutrition and food supplements can be obtained from a physician or hospital dietitian. (The hospital dietitian, incidentally, is a good person to know about—this staff member can be of great help to the patient and the patient's family in planning the proper nutrition for the person on treatment.)

Because lack of appetite is common with many cancer patients—particularly if they are undergoing chemotherapy or radiation—a high-protein-high-calorie food supplement may sometimes be required. Many pharmaceutical companies now are offering these supplements, which are often very helpful and come in various flavors such as vanilla, chocolate and butterscotch as well as in different forms: puddings, powders and milkshakes. Other supplements are flavorless and can be added to soups and fruit juices.

While a loss of appetite and difficulty in eating proper foods may be a problem for some cancer patients, more often patients who are receiving chemotherapy complain about gaining weight. Whether this is directly related to the chemicals themselves or because of nervousness that leads to excessive nibbling is not quite clear. In many situations the patient is able to go on a reasonable diet when the chemotherapy is completed, but it is not advisable for a patient to go on a crash diet while on chemotherapy.

It is important for family members and friends to encourage the patient to eat healthy meals—but not to use coercion if the patient does not particularly feel like eating. Coercion only leads to rebellion and frustration for all concerned.

Nonchemo-
therapeutic Drugs

While on chemotherapy, a patient can continue to take most medications such as minor tranquilizers, sleeping medication, pain killers and pills for high blood pressure, for the heart and for arthritis. However, a patient should not take any drugs that react negatively with such chemotherapeutic agents as Procarbazine or Matulane. It is also inadvisable to take aspirin, wonder drug though it may be, since aspirin interferes with clotting and may make bleeding problems worse. This would be a significant problem in patients whose platelet counts are very low (for example, below 100,000 and especially, below 50,000). Tylenol and Darvon are good substitutes for aspirin in cases of minor aches and pains. However, aspirin is not absolutely forbidden to patients undergoing chemotherapy who always have normal platelets.

A social drink is no problem—but this does not mean that a patient who has been undergoing intensive chemotherapy can consume six cans of beer in one evening. Patients who are taking Procarbazine or Matulane should not drink alcohol at all because of the adverse effect it has when combined with these medications.

In most instances cigarette smoking is not a difficult problem because many patients (and even their relatives) decide voluntarily to stop when treatment begins. Most physicians do recommend that a patient stop smoking if there is a chance for a long-term remission. In some cases where no such hope exists, the treatment goal may be just to make the patient as comfortable as possible. If giving up cigarettes would cause undue stress on such a patient, it might be better just to leave well enough alone and not to harass him or her about smoking. Ideally, the patient would stop smoking, but that decision depends on the patient, the cancer and the treatment.

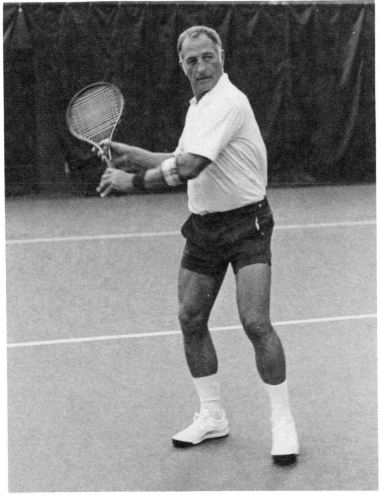

Many patients, like this man who had Hodgkin's disease, are able to continue their usual activities—including active sports—between chemotherapy treatments. His last treatment was in March, 1980.

Patients should continue to participate in any athletic activites they are accustomed to: jogging, bowling, golfing, tennis, swimming or whatever.

A case in point is a forty-five-year-old athletic coach who was diagnosed in April, 1976 as having Hodgkin's disease. A complete examination showed that it was still at a very early stage, and he was

Leisure and Recreation

treated with radiation. He was in complete remission until March, 1979, when he had a relapse and required vigorous chemotherapy. This patient was an avid tennis player and golfer. He requested that his treatments be given early in the week so that he would be well enough for his athletic activities on the weekends. His illness and treatment have caused only a minimal disruption of his active life-style and as of March, 1984, he was still in remission.

As with any activity, it is prudent for a cancer patient to participate in all athletic recreations as with anything else—in moderation.

Chemotherapy need not cancel travel and vacations. In fact, many patients can take long vacations (three or more months) while on chemotherapy. If a patient is going to be in a particular location for some length of time (say, residing in Florida during the winter), arrangements can be made for care by an oncologist in the community where the patient will be staying.

The American Cancer Society (ACS) and the Canadian Cancer Society (CCS) offer emotional as well as practical support for cancer patients.

The ACS sponsors a program in hospitals throughout the U.S. called I Can Cope. The program, which is free, helps patients learn about cancer and puts them in touch with other people in the same situation. Eight once-a-week meetings cover, among other things, understanding cancer, diagnosis, treatments, complications and self-care. Participants may include Cancer Society representatives, oncology nurses, social workers, physical therapists, dietitians, oncologists, lawyers and religious leaders.

The CCS has a similar, but smaller, program; call the local office of the CCS to get details. One program the CCS will tell you about is CanSurmount, a one-to-one visiting service in which a recovered cancer patient visits a newly-diagnosed cancer patient.

I Can Cope and similar groups offer a singular opportunity for group support, a sense of belonging, and knowledge that can greatly improve a patient's ability to cope with cancer on a day-to-day basis. Often, graduates of these programs continue to meet after the eight weeks are over. I urge cancer patients and their families to take advantage of I Can Cope or programs like it.

CHAPTER NINE

A Look Back and a Look Forward at a Hopeful Future

A history of cancer would involve looking back to classical times and would involve not only mankind, but the plant and animal kingdoms as well. Cancer has been found in such common plants as sunflowers and clover, and many of man's four-legged friends will benefit along with humans when the day comes that cancer is curable. Cancer is so common in mice, in fact, that mice are used with special frequency in certain experiments for cancer research.

Some kinds of cancer occur in specific racial groups; cancer of the liver appears with disproportionate frequency in the Bantus in some South African countries and in Malaysian people; a particular nasal-digestive cancer (of the nasopharynx) occurs at a high rate among the Chinese; and one kind of skin cancer almost never attacks black people. At first glance, it would appear that certain racial groups have genetic tendencies toward specific cancers, but researchers now suspect that environmental factors may also be at work in at least some of these mysteries. The frequency of stomach cancer among Icelanders, for example, which was once considered to have genetic origins, may instead be caused by hydrocarbons in the smoke used in curing fish. The high incidence of liver cancer in Africa may be due to a potent toxin caused by a fungus found in moldy peanuts.

Cancer research, to some extent, has been taking place ever since the days of the Greeks, but it started to come into its own as the microscope was perfected and scientists were able to hypothesize and later confirm that cancer is caused by abnormal cell division. The discovery that viruses might be involved in the origin of cancer occurred about 1910.

The Discovery of X Rays and Gamma Rays

Meanwhile, one of the most important advances in the battle against cancer had taken place in 1895: William Roentgen's discovery of X rays. Three years later Pierre and Marie Curie reported that some metallic elements, polonium, for example, gave off rays similar to X rays. Not long after, it was found that radium had this property, and the rays became known as *gamma rays*.

The next twenty years saw the production of reliable X ray equipment, and X ray beams could now be used for diagnosing and treating cancer. In 1900 the first radiotherapy for skin tumors was reported, and a year later radiotherapy for tumors deep inside the body took place. The great initial enthusiasm for the uses of X rays faded, however, when adverse effects began to show up—effects due principally to inadequate knowledge of proper doses, inadequate equipment, and lack of protection for both patients and therapists.

By 1930 safer equipment was available, and by that time protection and controls had been established. Furthermore, the medical profession now knew the correct doses and had learned that a single large dose could be replaced by smaller daily doses. By 1933 megavoltage, with its ability to penetrate tissue while sparing the skin, arrived on the scene. And in 1940, the betatron, forerunner of today's linear accelerators, was produced.

Chemotherapy Since the 1940s

Treatment of cancer was limited to surgery and radiation until chemotherapy came into use. Once the use of chemotherapy became common—not all that long ago—the history of cancer started to become a record of slow but increasing successes.

Chemotherapy has been used in the treatment of human cancer since the early 1940s, when nitrogen mustard was discovered to have an effect on lymph and blood cells. In 1942 chemotherapy involving nitrogen mustard was used to treat patients with cancer of the lymph system (malignant lymphoma) at Yale University in Connecticut. By 1945 nitrogen mustard chemotherapy was the firmly established practice for treating cancer of the lymph glands, and today nitrogen mustard is the foundation of the treatment of Hodgkin's disease.

In the early 1950s the drugs Busulfan and Chlorambucil were used to treat chronic leukemias. In the late '50s Cytoxan was discovered and has been used ever since to treat many types of cancer including leukemia, breast cancer, lung cancer and lymphomas such as Burkitt's lymphoma.

Great Success with Burkitt's Lymphoma

Burkitt's lymphoma is an unusual cancer found mostly among young children living in Africa in areas of high rainfall and humidity, where malaria is common. (However, it has no genetic or racial limitations, because it has also attacked children of European descent.) This cancer is unusual because it is probably the fastest-growing human cancer known, possibly doubling its size within twenty-four hours. Without appropriate treatment most patients would die of Burkitt's lymphoma within three months. Not only does this cancer affect the lymph glands and the bone, but it has also been known to attack any organ including the ovaries, kidneys, brain and, most frequently, the jaws. Burkitt's lymphoma attracted worldwide attention in medical circles when it was discovered to be associated with a virus (in this case the Epstein-Barr virus), and was found to be highly curable (80 percent if one excludes very advanced cases) with chemotherapy. It is reasonable to say that patients who are free of this disease after one year of treatment can probably be considered cured.

Importance of Methotrexate

Similar dramatic progress has been made in treating other types of cancer with chemotherapy. In 1949 another important chemotherapeutic drug, Methotrexate, was discovered. From the very beginning it provided great ammunition for the treatment of leukemias, but it was not until seven years later—in 1956—that its enormous value was truly recognized. For the first time a chemical agent could actually *cure* cancer. Methotrexate was found to produce complete remission in the treatment of a very rapidly spreading

107

tumor called choriocarcinoma, a cancer of the womb that occurs in women of child-bearing age.

Although rare in the United States, Canada and Europe, choriocarcinoma is common in Africa and Asia. It often appears as an abnormal pregnancy, although occasionally it may be associated with a normal pregnancy or may appear soon after a normal delivery. Its symptoms are a rapidly enlarging womb, profuse vaginal bleeding that may lead to anemia, and excessive nausea and vomiting. The cancer tends to spread rapidly from the womb to other parts of the body, especially the lungs. Before chemotherapy, total or partial

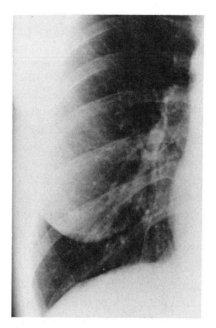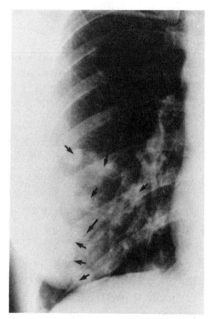

Complete response of choriocarcinoma to chemotherapy. In the X ray at left, arrows point to cancerous white lumps where the cancer had spread to the lung area. The lumps are gone in the X ray at right. (Courtesy of Mostafa Selim, M.D.)

removal of the womb (hysterectomy) was the main treatment, which provided less than a 2 percent survival rate among patients with metastasis. Even if the tumor did not spread and a total hysterectomy was performed, the survival rate was still only 40 percent.

In 1956, two physicians produced a spectacular response in three patients with choriocarcinoma by treating them with Methotrexate.

This was the first time that chemotherapy had been shown to produce a complete disappearance of cancer. In 1960, Actinomycin D was used in combination with Methotrexate and resulted in a 75 percent rate of cure. Now over 90 percent of all patients with choriocarcinoma, including women who have lung metastasis, can be cured. This combination chemotherapy results in virtually 100 percent cure in cases where the tumor is localized in the womb. This cancer produces HGC—human chorionic gonadotropin—hormones, and by performing simple blood tests for HCG levels in the body, a physician can tell with extreme accuracy when all the cancer cells have been eradicated and when chemotherapy can be ended. In most cases there is no need for a hysterectomy, so young patients who are cured with chemotherapy can have normal pregnancies and deliveries.

The next landmark in chemotherapy was the discovery that significant rates of cure could result from the use of several drugs in combination. Not only did this mean progress in the treatment of rare diseases like choriocarcinoma with Actimomycin D and Methotrexate, but it also meant great progress in the treatment of more common types of cancer. Hodgkin's disease is an example. Researchers discovered relatively early that one drug produced a 30 percent remission in Hodgkin's disease, and with two the effectiveness doubled. However, the duration of the benefit from the two chemicals was still quite short. Later, in the mid-1960s, it was discovered that the combined use of the four chemicals together known as MOPP could produce a rate of cure as high as 70 to 80 percent, even when the Hodgkin's disease had reached advanced stages. Equally significant achievements occurred in the mid-1970s with the treatment of testicular cancer, which once had a high mortality rate in young men in their twenties and early thirties. Now the use of a combination of drugs results in an almost 100 percent rate of cure in moderately advanced cases of some forms of testicular cancers, and 70 percent is possible even at advanced stages of the disease. Likewise, the treatment of breast cancer was improved in the 1970s with the use of combination chemotherapy, especially when the drugs were given soon after surgery to patients with an early spread of the tumor. And in certain acute leukemias in children, combination chemotherapy results in cures in about 80 percent of the cases.

Discovery of Combination Chemotherapy

The chemotherapeutic drugs developed since the 1940s for the treatment of cancer were discovered after extensive research. Some of the drugs were synthesized in the laboratory or purified from plant products, and others are antibiotics made from bacteria. For every chemotherapeutic drug that finally becomes available to the public, probably 100 similar compounds have been manufactured, tested in animals and then rejected as unsuitable for humans. Only the compounds that have been tested repeatedly and are found to be effective and reasonably safe are approved for general use. This is why, after over forty years of research and experimentation, only approximately three dozen chemicals are available for general use in the treatment of cancer.

Causes of Cancer
The outlook for future progress in the treatment of cancer appears quite hopeful. Nearly 50 percent of all cancers now diagnosed are curable. Although the major causes of cancers are not known, it has been clearly demonstrated that environmental factors and personal habits have been linked to some forms of cancer. By and large, lung cancer is due to smoking, making lung cancer a preventable disease. In fact, 20 percent of *all* cancers can be linked to smoking. There is no effective means of early detection for lung cancer as yet, nor are there effective methods of controlling lung cancer in the majority of cases, once it is detected. About 25 percent of all cancer deaths are now cases of lung cancer. Prevention, therefore, must be the cornerstone of the efforts used to control this and other cancers caused by personal habits.

Oncogenes and
Oncoviruses
Other significant causes of cancer are now beginning to emerge—specifically, genes and viruses. Knowledge of the exact mechanism whereby genes and viruses cause cancer will be of enormous help in future prevention and treatment of many cancers. *Genes* are the units within our bodies that control the development of inherited traits. Genes that cause cancer are called *oncogenes*. These genes, a normal part of the animal and human inheritance system, are essential in the body's early development, after which they stop functioning.

Oncogenes can go into a dormant stage during later life—an

inactive state in which they are called *protooncogenes*. On the other hand, they can be reactivated, again becoming oncogenes, having been "turned on" by a wide variety of environmental stimuli such as radiation, cancer-causing chemicals, viruses and other stimuli not yet known.

Oncogenes, which are found in less than 20 percent of cancers studied, have been discovered in colon, lung, muscle and bladder cancers. The same oncogenes can be found in extremely different types of tumors; on the other hand, different oncogenes have been found in the same type of cancer in different patients. Clearly, further understanding of oncogenes may explain why normal cells become malignant and, most importantly, how this could be prevented or terminated.

A *virus* is any one of various disease-causing agents that can reproduce themselves only inside a living cell. *Oncoviruses* are cancer-causing viruses. It has been well established for many decades that viruses play an especially significant role in causing such cancers as leukemia and lymph-system cancers in animals. It has long been suspected—but never proved—that viruses may be a factor in human cancer. The Epstein-Barr virus (EBV) has been associated with Burkitt's lymphoma as well as with cancers of the nose and pharynx. EBV is also associated with lymphomas in transplant patients whose resistance is very low.

It was not until 1980 that Dr. Robert C. Gallo proved the existence of a virus that can cause human leukemia. He isolated for the first time the *human T-cell leukemia virus* (HTLV). HTLV causes certain leukemias and lymphomas that are most commonly found in Japan and the Caribbean, although cases have also turned up in the United States, Israel, Africa and South America.

The Link Between Viruses and Human Cancer

In laboratory studies, HTLV can turn human bone-marrow cells and blood cells into cancerous cells. The leukemia or lymphoma caused by HTLV occurs in adults in early middle age, usually follows an acute course, and often is associated with high blood calcium and extensive bone destruction.

The exact method of transmission of HTLV is not fully known, but it is probably spread by insects or blood products. This virus is not particularly contagious and in order to spread may require prolonged close contact in order for one person to get the disease from another. It may even take up to twenty years between the time of contact and the time the disease manifests itself. Not everyone who has HTLV develops cancer. There may be some genetic predisposition to contracting the disease.

Some people develop antibodies to the virus that protect them from getting the disease. On the other hand, some patients with antibodies are not protected, and some people are unable to produce sufficient antibodies and are more susceptible.

The researchers working with Dr. Gallo have recently isolated a virus very similar to the original HTLV that they have labelled HTLV II. They suspect that both HTLVs may be associated with or cause more cancers than are known now. In fact, some authorities speculate that these viruses may be the cause of, or be associated with, AIDS. It is possible that vaccines or other methods of immunization could some day be used to prevent cancers due to HTLV.

How AIDS May Help Solve Cancer Mysteries

Acquired Immune Deficiency Syndrome (AIDS) provides a fruitful area for cancer research. A strong link exists among AIDS, cancer, immune deficiency, viruses and certain lifestyles. Of the approximately 5,000 cases of AIDS reported in the United States, 70 percent are homosexual males, 17 percent are drug abusers and 1 percent are hemophiliacs. Of the remaining cases, about 150 are not considered to come from any of the high-risk groups, but some of these 150 may be heterosexual sex partners of AIDS patients. Most cases in the U.S. are in New York, which has 50 percent of the cases, and in San Francisco and Miami. Of the twenty other nations that have reported patients with AIDS, less than 200 documented cases are known.

AIDS patients have defective immune systems that make them highly susceptible to infections by "opportunistic" organisms—those that normally attack only seriously ill and debilitated patients. AIDS patients also have a very high incidence of a unique cancer called Kaposi's sarcoma—and they have a particularly virulent form of it.

Kaposi's Sarcoma

Kaposi's sarcoma has been found in about 33 percent of AIDS patients. The typical Kaposi's sarcoma is common in some parts of

Africa and in the Mediterranean basin, but is very rare in the United States, where only about 100 cases are reported annually. It attacks people over the age of sixty and usually appears on the legs as numerous purplish nodules that contain large numbers of blood vessels. This cancer is treatable and rarely causes early death. Survival is usually ten to fifteen years from onset of the disease, with many of the victims eventually dying of other causes.

The Kaposi's sarcoma associated with AIDS is quite different, occurring in previously healthy young people. It is a more aggressive disease that is diffuse, rather than restricted to a specific area, and may involve generalized lymph-node enlargement as well as internal organs such as the liver and spleen. It is also associated with a high death rate, the average survival being only fifteen months, in contrast to fifteen years for the typical Kaposi's sarcoma. Some patients in high-risk AIDS groups have developed persistent generalized lymph-node enlargement along with laboratory evidence of immune deficiency—but they do not have other clinical evidence of AIDS such as fever, fatigue, weight loss, night sweats and infections.

Unlike healthy homosexual males, the majority of homosexual AIDS patients have engaged in sexual encounters with hundreds of different sexual partners—often a lifetime average of over 1,000 different partners. As a consequence, many of these men have been infected by numerous sexually transmitted diseases. Drug addicts are also prone to numerous infections because they have used contaminated drugs and needles. Both these groups can exhaust their immune systems because of persistent frequent infections. People with severe hemophilia are another group that is exposed to frequent infections and foreign antigens. (Antigens cause the production of antibodies; repeated demands on the antibodies could result in the exhaustion of the immune system).* Furthermore, a medication commonly used by hemophiliacs is pooled from the plasma of 2,000 to 5,000 donors, resulting in a high incidence of blood-transmitted viruses. The use of a different anti-hemophilia concentrate (such as cryoprecipitate, which is pooled from the blood of about fifteen to twenty donors), could significantly reduce blood-transmitted infec-

Exhausted Immune Systems in AIDS Victims

*Antigens are discussed later in this chapter in the section on monoclonal antibodies.

tions in hemophilic patients. Although it appears that AIDS can be transmitted through certain blood components during a transfusion, this method of infection is extremely rare. Annually only about ten cases of AIDS are reported in the U.S. in which there could be any possible link to over 10 million transfusions.

Possible Causes and Prevention of AIDS

Different viruses have been implicated as the cause of AIDS. Recently, the human T-cell leukemia virus (referred to in the preceding section on oncoviruses) has been regarded as the most likely candidate. Virus and antibody studies support linkage of HTLV and AIDS. If AIDS is transmitted by infectious agents, it is definitely not very contagious.

It is now clear that AIDS affects only people with immune defects, although possibly other genetic and environmental factors may also be involved. The incubation period—the time from acquiring the disease to the time the victim is aware of it—is approximately twelve to eighteen months, but it can be as short as six months or as long as five years.

In summary, it is clear that AIDS is not a disease that attacks healthy people unless they have some predisposing immune suppression. Nor is it acquired by casual contact with AIDS patients. The chances of developing AIDS from a random blood transfusion are minuscule—probably less than one in a million. Therefore to designate AIDS as an epidemic, or to fear contracting AIDS from a blood transfusion or blood donation, or from restaurants that homosexuals frequent, is unfounded.

Although much has been learned about AIDS in the short time since its discovery in 1979, there is as yet no satisfactory treatment for it. Preventive steps remain the best approach. These include:

- Avoiding persistent sexual contact with high-risk people;
- Limiting the number of sexual partners if one is a male homosexual;
- Avoiding the use of contaminated drugs and shared needles;
- Seeing to it, if one is in a position to, that people in high risk groups do not donate blood.

Since cancer may be due to a great extent to a breakdown in the body's immunity, and to a small extent to viruses, any new knowledge regarding the cause, treatment and prevention of AIDS may be of great value in the treatment of cancer.

114

If the exact cause of AIDS is confirmed as a specific virus, possibly a vaccine and/or antibodies could be developed to treat or prevent it.

Early detection will continue to be very important in the fight against cancer. It is the fervent hope of the medical profession that if patients are aware of how much can now be done for them they will seek early and, most important, *proper* help. The routine use of the Pap test for women has helped to reduce substantially the scourge of cervical cancer. Self-examination for breast and testicular cancers should be encouraged, since both of these are usually curable at early stages. Colon and rectal cancers (which are among the leading cancers in the western hemisphere), can be diagnosed early through detection of blood in the stool, an inexpensive procedure that should be done one or two times a year for people over forty.

Early Diagnosis— Still the Best Weapon

Some cancers produce chemicals that can be detected in the blood. Common examples include *CEA* in colon cancer, *HCG* in some uterine and testicular cancers, and *LDH* in many other cancers, especially lymph-system cancers. When these chemicals appear in tests, they often signify advanced disease. Therefore the tests for these chemicals need to be more refined and specific. There is a definite need for discovery of new and more sensitive cancer-indicating chemicals, and research is now under way to find them. It will be a wonderful day when such tests can be done inexpensively and accurately to screen patients with very early cancers.

The Search for Cancer-Indicating Chemicals in Blood

Two of the newer diagnostic tools that are very helpful in the early detection of cancer are *ultrasound* and the *CAT scan*. Ultrasound is a special device that makes images through the transmission of sound waves; the CAT scan is a very sensitive computer scan. Both techniques are especially useful in the diagnosis of such cancers as ovarian cancer and lymphoma of the abdomen, because in many instances the only other means of discovering these tumors would be exploratory surgery. Ultrasound and CAT scans are valuable not only in diagnosis but also later on, once treatment has started, because they can indicate what is happening to the cancer.

Ultrasound and CAT Scans

One of the newest diagnostic techniques is *nuclear magnetic resonance (NMR)*. This makes it possible for a physician to know what's happening inside the body without the use of surgery or radiation. Overall, NMR is not superior to a CAT scan but, rather, complements it. However, in some situations NMR is better than a CAT scan—particularly in examining the posterior, the lower brain, and the spinal cord and in detection of early prostate cancer.

The use of *laser beams* in cancer surgery may make it possible for surgeons to operate easily on parts of the body that are relatively inaccessible by conventional means. Lasers, by converting electromagnetic energy into intensely concentrated light energy, can be directed very precisely and can literally melt tumors away while sparing the surrounding normal tissues.

LASER stands for Light Amplification by Stimulated Emission of Radiation. Electrical energy passes through a tube containing lasing material such as carbon dioxide or argon, where the atoms become agitated. These agitated atoms emit light waves that can be concentrated through a special mirror. The lasing material determines the beam's depth of penetration and the wave length, which in turn determines what will absorb the laser beam. The laser beam can be focused with great precision—up to a fraction of a millimeter—to eliminate cancerous tissue only.

Laser surgery can be performed without any pulling or tearing; in the brain, for example, a tumor can be neatly destroyed with only minimal trauma or damage to the surrounding normal tissue. Some types of laser energy, in order to destroy tumors at inaccessible locations, can even be transmitted through flexible optical instruments. This technique in an expert's hands is very useful in treating hard-to-reach esophageal or bronchial tumors or bladder tumors that are causing bleeding or obstruction. This can lead to immediate relief in swallowing, breathing, or urinating. Since one effect of laser energy is to eliminate bleeding, healing after laser surgery is fairly prompt, with minimal bleeding or scar formation. Most laser surgery can be done on an outpatient basis.

An area of treatment that is not new, but in which there has been steady progress, is the use of radiation. The search now is for radiation energy that will destroy cancer cells and leave surrounding normal cells intact. Experiments have resulted in the successful use of high-energy radiation such as the "fast neutrons" that are giving improved results in radiation (see Chapter 4). Today, various types of radiation therapies that are either in use or in the research stage include X rays, gamma rays, cobalt therapy, electron beams, neutrons and pi mesons, which oncologists in the future will be able to use in combination, as they have done with drugs in chemotherapy. This may well improve radiation results and reduce any side effects. Combinations of radiation and surgery could lead to improvement in the treatment of some cancers that are presently inoperable.

A major goal for the future is increasing the body's defense mechanisms to eliminate residual cancer cells. While today's conventional treatments for cancer can eliminate the bulk of a tumor, we still need ways of stimulating the immunological system. This could be very useful in preventing a return of a cancer. Here *interferon* may play an important role. This is a protein known, ever since it was first described around the mid-1960s, to have anti-virus properties. Since the mid-'70s it has also been shown to have an effect on cancer in studies done mainly in Switzerland and in the Scandinavian countries, especially in Sweden. Interferon increases the body's ability to attack viruses and also cancer cells. There is some evidence that it may also be able, like radiation or chemotherapy, to act directly on the cancer cells by interfering with cell division.

Increasing the Body's Defenses with Interferon

Interferon has been reported to be useful in treating a wide variety of cancers—for example, leukemias, Hodgkin's disease, breast cancer and bone cancers such as osteogenic sarcoma or multiple myeloma. In many of these cases, however, the remissions were incomplete or the disease was stabilized for only a short time. Interferon, as we know it today, has *not* produced cures and is not the miracle drug it has been reported to be. It is unfortunate that unusually high expectations have been generated about interferon by the news media, drug companies, and a few researchers.

There is no doubt that interferon will probably some day produce beneficial effects and become a very useful tool in the fight against

Interferon in Experimental Stage

cancer, especially if it is used in conjunction with other methods of treatment. At this point, a major part of researchers' efforts should be spent in producing interferon in pure form. (At present the protein given as interferon contains only about 1 percent pure interferon.) Many of the unpleasant side effects such as fever, chills, muscle aches, weight loss, and hair loss are probably due to protein impurities. If the interferon content of the protein mixture could be substantially increased, the response rate in cancer treatment might be raised proportionately. However, as of 1984 it must be emphasized that interferon is at the experimental stage and there is no definite evidence that it can by itself cure cancer. It is premature for patients to stop conventional treatments and assume that interferon is all they need.

The Promise of Monoclonal Antibodies

Among all the discoveries in immunotherapy to date, *monoclonal antibodies* may hold the greatest promise. Monoclonal antibodies may be the dream, the magic bullet that can be directed selectively against malignant cells or other disease-causing organisms.

The basic immunological process the body uses to defend itself against foreign or abnormal elements such as viruses, bacteria, cancer or anything else is the interaction between *antigens* and *antibodies*. Antigens are proteins or chemical particles located on the cells. The antigens on disease-causing organisms trigger other, specialized cells to produce proteins called antibodies. The antibodies track down and damage or kill the disease-causing agents. Antibodies, which are produced by special white blood cells, are Y-shaped molecules that fit the antigens as precisely as a key fits a lock. Normally, an invading organism with numerous antigens on its cell walls may trigger random production of thousands of antibodies called polyclonal (having many clones) antibodies. Only a few of these polyclonal antibodies are necessary (or are produced in sufficient quantities) to kill the offending organisms. When a sufficient number of antibodies attach themselves to the antigens on a cell wall, a series of chemical reactions takes place, leading to the rupture of the cell wall and the death of the targeted cell.

The First Monoclonals

For decades researchers have been trying to produce large quantities of a highly purified single, specialized antibody that could be directed against a specific antigen. In 1975 two scientists in England succeeded; they devised a method of producing a single antibody called a monoclonal antibody. They selected two unique cells and fused them into a single cell, a unique hybrid cell capable of producing pure antibodies and also of growing and dividing *indefinitely*.

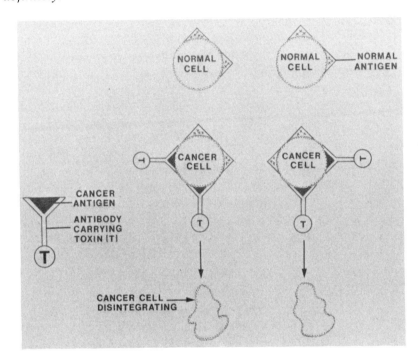

Monoclonal antibodies—potential magic bullets. A toxin (*T*) attached to a monoclonal antibody tracks down the antigen on cancer cells and destroys those cells while leaving normal antigens and normal cells intact.

The most common method of producing monoclonal antibodies at present is as follows:

1. A selected cell with special antigens is injected into a mouse. This causes certain white blood cells (lymphocytes) in the mouse's spleen to start producing antibodies.
2. The mouse's spleen is then removed and the special antibody-producing white cells are isolated—"harvested"—from the spleen.

3. These spleen cells are fused with myeloma (bone cancer) cells. The hybrid cells, which are cancerous and have the ability to produce antibodies, are called hybridoma, an abbreviated form of hybrid myeloma.

4. At this stage there are many hybridomas, all of which are capable of producing different antibodies. The hybridomas are separated according to the type of antibodies produced. This is called cloning.

5. Each clone of hybridomas is now capable of producing a specific type of antibody. These clones can be cultured in the laboratory to divide forever and produce large quantities of pure antibodies, or they can be stored indefinitely in a freezer to be used as needed. These clones, when injected into the abdominal cavity of a mouse, can propagate and produce large quantities of monoclonal antibodies.

This system of producing monoclonal antibodies is very slow and tedious, and takes several months. Even though the potential uses of monoclonal antibodies are almost unlimited, their use as a weapon against cancer on a large scale is still at an early stage.

Nevertheless, specific monoclonal antibodies are now available for brain, breast, and colon cancers as well as lymphoma, leukemia and melonoma. Even though there have been a few impressive reports of complete disappearances of cancers treated with monoclonal antibodies, these are still the exceptions. Monoclonal antibodies could be used in the future as carriers of chemotherapeutic drugs, highly selective radiation, or even toxins to selectively attack cancer cells and spare normal cells. Preliminary work has shown that a diphtheria toxin bound to a mouse's monoclonal antibody can selectively kill human colon cancer.

Monoclonals in Diagnosing and Locating Tumors
One of the most important potential uses of monoclonals is in the rapid diagnosis of cancer as well as finding its starting point. Occasionally a tumor may be extremely difficult to diagnose after a biopsy is taken, and sometimes a number of independent experts will each have different opinions regarding the diagnosis. For proper treatment, cancer must be diagnosed accurately. Staining the biopsy specimen with a panel of monoclonal antibodies could result in rapid and accurate diagnosis of these difficult cases.

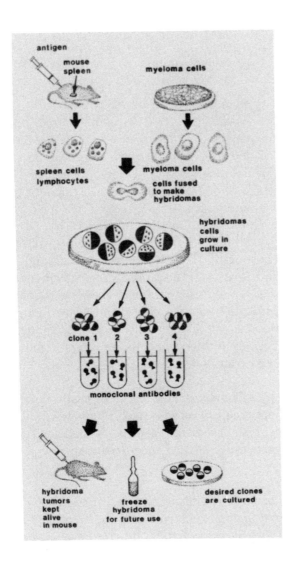

Often a patient may have early or advanced metastatic cancer, but the primary cancer itself will be very difficult to find. The search for the primary cancer can be laborious, expensive and often painful. Potentially, the injection of monoclonal antibodies could solve this problem and eliminate the need for much exploratory surgery. In other cases, a small biopsy sample taken by a needle is sometimes too small for an accurate diagnosis; staining the tiny biopsy sample with monoclonals could clarify the diagnosis and, again, eliminate another biopsy or exploratory surgery.

Other Uses
of Monoclonals

The staging of cancer—determining whether it is in an early or advanced stage—is very important in treatment; for example, lymph-node involvement in breast cancer may determine whether additional treatment is needed after surgery. In the future, an oncologist could inject monoclonal antibodies into the lymph system of the breast or other organs and outline exactly the extent of lymph-node metastasis.

Monoclonal antibodies could be one of the most versatile and significant developments of modern medicine. They may turn out to be especially useful in the rapid and accurate measurement of enzymes and hormones. Their use in the diagnosis and treatment of early hormone disorders and infections, especially in cancer patients, is one of the possibilities being explored. They may become extremely useful in purification of chemicals and compounds, especially interferon. Monoclonals are already becoming valuable in blood banking—especially in blood and tissue typing—and in aiding in transfusions and transplants, which are very important in cancer treatment.

Because hybridomas are able to mutate easily, it will be possible to develop mutants capable of selectively binding and killing different kinds of cancer cells. The potential uses of monoclonal antibodies to be fully explored, especially in cancer treatment, are countless.

The Continuing
Importance of
Chemotherapy

In spite of these promising new advances, chemotherapy will continue to play an important role in cancer treatment in the future. One major branch of research today is in the development of drugs to control the side effects of chemotherapy; for example, there are now three different medications that can prevent severe nausea and vomiting caused by Cisplatinum. In addition, significant new drugs will be developed to attack cancer cells. These new drugs, and the more effective use of current ones, should inevitably lead to better results.

A Guide to
Chemotherapeutic Drugs

The following is a list of the most frequently used chemotherapeutic drugs (or chemotherapeutic agents). Each description includes the types of cancers the drug is used against, how the drug is given and any side effects. Although some of the side effects may sound alarming, severe side effects are actually very rare; most patients experience only mild to moderate side effects, some none at all. Also, remember that most side effects can be prevented or treated (see Chapter 7). I urge patients who experience any discomfort to tell their physicians. Suffering in silence is unnecessary.

Actinomycin D. (See **D-Actinomycin.**)

Adriamycin. This drug is made from antibiotics and is very effective against breast cancer, lymph-system cancer, acute leukemia, soft-tissue tumors (sarcomas), and some lung tumors. It is given only intravenously, and its side effects, which can be quite severe, include severe irritation and inflammation of the skin and muscle tissue if the needle is not securely in the vein. Patients who experience any pain or redness at the IV injection area should call a doctor or nurse immediately. The heart muscles may be affected when the total dose approaches 800 to 1,000 mg., a level that may be reached after about eight to twelve months of treatment. In elderly patients the dose becomes dangerous at a much lower level, particularly in those who already have heart problems. However, heart problems brought on by use of Adriamycin occur very rarely because they can usually be avoided by a careful watch over the total dose as well as by frequent cardiac examinations and EKGs. A simple but sensitive test called a Muga scan, which measures heart-muscle strength, can help avoid serious problems. Occasionally, red urine (which should be carefully distinguished from blood in the urine) may be noticed. Hair loss is quite common, particularly if Adriamycin is used in combination with other drugs such as Oncovin.

Alkeran. (See **Melphalan.**)

BCNU. (See **Nitrosoureas.**)

Busulfan (Myleran). Busulfan is the first line of defense against chronic myelogenous leukemia and, in rare cases, may be used against cancers of the ovary and breast. It is given as a pill, and its side effects include skin changes such as deeper color or, in isolated cases, hives. Occasionally, after very prolonged treatment, inflammation of the lung can develop, which can be serious.

CCNU. (See **Nitrosoureas.**)

Chlorambucil (Leukeran). Chlorambucil is effective in the treatment of chronic lymphatic leukemias and is moderately effective against tumors of the ovary, breast and testicles. Chlorambucil is given as a pill. Its side effects are mild and include slight nausea and a slight to moderate drop in blood count, depending on the dose and how long it is given.

Cisplatinum (Platinol). Effective against a wide range of cancers including tumors of the testicles, ovaries, head and neck, lung, and lymph system, Cisplatinum is usually given over several hours as a slow intravenous infusion. The preferred method of treatment is on an inpatient basis because of severe nausea and vomiting as side effects. Some loss of hearing as well as kidney damage (which can be prevented by vigorous hydration), can also be major side effects.

Cosmegen. (See **D-Actinomycin.**)

Cyclophosphamide (Cytoxan). This drug is useful against a wide variety of tumors, especially multiple myelomas (bone tumors) and cancers of the lymph system, breast, ovary, and lung. It can be given as a pill or intravenously and can cause nausea, vomiting, and hair loss. Large doses can result in irritation and inflammation of the bladder and result in blood in the urine. In moderate doses, however, this side effect is rare. Adequate hydration is required to prevent cystitis (the inflammation of the bladder that causes blood in the urine).

Cytosinearabinoside (Cytosar). Although this drug has very limited use, it is particularly effective in the treatment of acute leukemias and, occasionally, lymph-system cancer. It can be injected under the skin or into a vein. Side effects are nausea, vomiting and a low blood count.

Cytoxan. (See **Cyclophosphamide.**)

D-Actinomycin (Actinomycin D, Cosmegen). D-Actinomycin is used in the treatment of soft-tissue tumors as well as tumors of the testicles and uterus. It is also effective in the treatment of two childhood tumors: Wilm's tumors and neuroblastoma. Given only intravenously by slow infusion, it can cause severe nausea, vomiting, hair loss, a severe drop in blood count and irritation or inflammation at the area of infusion if it happens to leak out of the vein.

Daunomycin (Daunorubicin). This is a sister medication of Adriamycin; they come from the same antibiotics and there is only a slight chemical difference between them. Adriamycin, however, is widely used, while Daunomycin is used almost exclusively in the treatment of acute leukemias. Daunomycin, like Adriamycin, is given intravenously and has similar side effects.

Depo Provera. Used in the treatment of ovarian and endometrial cancers as well as cancer of the kidney, Depo Provera is given as an intramuscular injection, and is usually used in combination with other drugs. There are only minimal side effects, which include fluid retention, and it can aggravate diabetes and hypertension.

Dicarbazine (DTIC). Dicarbazine is useful in the treatment of leukemia, lymph-system cancer and skin tumors known as melanomas. It is given only intravenously by drip infusion. The side effects are usually severe nausea and vomiting, which can last over several hours. It can cause flulike discomfort, with muscle aches and headaches, or a lowered blood count, lasting two to four weeks after treatment, which is why blood count is watched very closely.

DTIC (See **Dicarbazine,** above.)

Etoposide. (See **VP 16.**)

5-FU (5-Fluorouracil). This drug is used mostly for cancer of the breast, stomach and colon. When a bowel tumor has spread to the liver, 5-FU can be given by a special technique (called *hepatic artery infusion*) in which 5-FU is injected directly into the liver. It is usually used in combination with other drugs. Side effects include nausea and vomiting, which are usually mild unless a large dose is given. Hair loss is slight, and occasionally there is a darkening of the skin, particularly in the area where the needle is inserted. Dryness or thinning of the skin, or an occasional rash, may also occur. But except for mild nausea, these side effects are extremely rare.

Halotestin. Useful in the treatment of breast cancer as well as in stimulating the production of new blood, Halotestin is always given as a pill. Because it is a male hormone, it causes mild to heavy facial-hair growth, especially if used over a long period of time. It can also cause mild to severe liver damage, which may be reversible, and sometimes results in fluid retention.

Hydroxyurea (Hydrea). Hydroxyurea is useful in the treatment of a particular form of chronic leukemia, and also has a mild effect on cancer of the kidney and colon. It is given as a pill. Because it can cause a very rapid drop in the blood count of leukemia patients if large doses are given, the blood count is watched very closely.

Hydrea. (See **Hydroxyurea,** above.)

L-Asparaginase. This is one of the few known chemicals that can prevent tumor cells from getting certain nutrients essential to cancer cells but not required by normal cells. (One of these nutrients is L-asparagine, an amino acid.) L-Asparaginase is very useful in the treatment of acute lymphoblastic leukemias, especially in children. The drug is given slowly (over at least two hours) by intravenous injection. It is advisable that the patient be hospitalized; if the patient is treated on an outpatient basis, the physician should be contacted immediately if there is the slightest problem. L-Asparaginase has many side effects, some of which are potentially dangerous. The major difficulties are allergic reaction, fever and inflammation of the pancreas, which can result in severe abdominal pain and even shock.

Leukeran. (See **Chlorambucil.**)

Melphalan (Alkeran). Melphalan is useful principally in treating breast and ovarian cancers and multiple myeloma (bone cancer that is in several locations). It is usually given as a pill, although in rare cases may be given intravenously. Side effects are usually limited to mild nausea, but large doses and prolonged treatment can cause a severe drop in blood count.

Methotrexate. Methotrexate is useful against leukemia, lymphomas, breast tumors, uterine tumors (choriocarcinoma) and tumors of the head, neck and bladder. It can be given both orally and intravenously, and is particularly effective in treating spinal leukemia when injected directly into the spinal fluid. Side effects may include a severe decrease in the blood count, a sore mouth and diarrhea. The kidneys, liver and lungs could be affected if large doses are given or if treatment is prolonged. Methotrexate is the only chemotherapeutic drug that has an antidote. This allows very high doses to be given, and, about twenty-four hours after the patient takes the drug, the antidote (folinic acid) can be taken to block the side effects. The beneficial aspects of the drug are unaffected by the antidote.

Myleran. (See **Busulfan.**)

Nitrosoureas (BCNU, CCNU). This is a group of drugs that includes BCNU and CCNU and is effective against brain tumors, colon cancers, Hodgkin's disease, bone cancer and lymph-system cancer. They can be given either orally or intravenously. If BCNU is given by intravenous injection, it must be diluted and given by slow infusion because otherwise it would cause severe pain and burning along the vein. Nitrosoureas can cause severe nausea, vomiting and prolonged low blood count (lasting as long as six weeks).

Nolvadex. (See **Tamoxifen.**)

Oncovin. (See **Vincristine.**)

Platinol. (See **Cisplatinum.**)

Prednisone. Prednisone is a steroid capable of destroying malignant white blood cells called lymphocytes. It is useful in treating Hodgkin's disease, leukemias, and certain bone cancers (multiple myeloma), as well as the side effects of brain metastasis or brain tumors. It is also helpful in reducing the high calcium level in the blood that bone tumors can cause. Prednisone is given in the form of a pill; in order to avoid long-lasting side effects, it is given intermittently—with "time off" during the treatment. Prednisone has many side effects, some of which can be quite severe, but these usually occur only when the doses are large and are given over a long period of time. Side effects can range from acid stomach to ulcers to mental changes (with depression being the most likely). There can be a marked increase in appetite. If the patient has diabetes, Prednisone may make it worse, and if latent diabetes exists, the Prednisone may cause it to appear. Long-term use of Prednisone (or any other steroid) can lead to weakened bones and muscles.

6 MP (6-Mercaptopurine). Almost the only use of 6 MP is in the treatment of acute leukemias. It is given as a pill, and side effects usually include mild nausea and vomiting. Large doses can cause severe mouth ulcers and lowered blood count. In rare cases, it causes liver damge (which is usually reversible). When combined with Zyloprim, the dosage of 6 MP is reduced because Zyloprim keeps 6 MP in the blood longer, which could lead to an increase of side effects.

Tamoxifen (Nolvadex). Tamoxifen is particularly effective in women who have breast tumors that depend on estrogen or female hormones. It is taken orally and is unique because its side effects are minimal: mild vaginal discharge, mild nausea and hot flashes that are usually only temporary. Very prolonged use can aggravate cataracts of the eyes, so regular eye examinations are recommended for patients who have cataracts.

Vinblastine (Velban). This drug, which comes from the periwinkle plant, is a major part of the treatment of Hodgkin's disease and testicular cancers. Breast cancers and lymphomas are also responsive to it. It is only given intravenously because the body does not absorb it well in pill form. Almost always used in combination with other chemotherapeutic drugs, Vinblastine must be given with care so it will not filter into the tissues. It can cause low blood count, mild numbness, tingling in the extremities and mild constipation.

Vincristine (Oncovin). Vincristine was discovered about the same time, and comes from the same plant, as Vinblastine. Its major advantage is that it neither affects nor reduces the blood count; in fact, it may increase the platelet count. It is used against Hodgkin's disease, lymphomas, breast tumors, leukemias, and childhood leukemias such as Wilm's tumor, with results ranging from very effective to moderately effective. As with Vinblastine, it is given intravenously with special care to make sure it does not filter into the tissues. Its most common side effects include temporary nerve impairment, which causes numbness, tingling and weakness in the hands and feet, and is reversible. Constipation can occur, and can be severe unless the proper precautions are taken. Jaw pain and, in rare cases, fever can also occur. These side effects are much more severe than those of Vinblastine.

VP16 (Etoposide). VP16, which is a plant product, is a new drug, released for general use in 1984. VP16 may turn out to be the most important drug yet in the treatment of small-cell cancer of the lung. When used alone, it produces about 50 percent response, but it is more often used in combination with other drugs. It also has some effect on some leukemias and lymph-system cancers. Side effects include a blood count that will be especially low in white cells; nausea and vomiting; and hair loss (which will not last). Allergic reactions such as fever, chills and wheezing may occur and can be easily treated with antihistamines. Occasionally hypotension (low blood pressure) occurs, which can usually be corrected by slowing down the infusion rate.

Glossary

Words That Will Be Useful in Talking
with Health-Care Professionals

This list includes specialized words used in this book as well as a few that have not been but that might come up in discussions.

ADENOCARCINOMA. Cancer in gland-forming tissues such as those of the breast, lung or gastrointestinal tract.

ADJUVANT TREATMENT. Additional treatment (for example, radiation or chemotherapy after surgery).

ANEMIA. A deficiency of red blood cells, which carry oxygen.

ANTI-HORMONES. Chemotherapeutic drugs that work by blocking certain hormones that are known to stimulate the growth of some cancers.

ARTERY. A blood vessel that carries oxygen-rich blood *from* the heart to the tissues. (See also *vein.*)

BENIGN. Noncancerous, nonmalignant.

BIOPSY. Surgical removal of tissue for examination and diagnosis.

BLOOD COUNT. The number of red cells and white cells and platelets in a blood sample.

BONE MARROW. The soft inner part of the bone where blood cells are made.

CANCER. A malignant growth or tumor. (*Cancer* and *tumor* are used interchangeably in this book).

CARCINOMA. Cancer or a form of cancer.

CAT SCAN. A very sensitive three-dimensional computer scan able to detect minute tumors and abnormalities in the body. (CAT stands for Computer Assisted Tomography.)

CELL. The smallest unit of the body.

CHEMOTHERAPY. The treatment of cancer using chemicals or drugs. These chemicals are referred to as *chemotherapeutic drugs* or *chemotherapeutic agents.*

CHROMOSOMES. Threads of material located in the central part of the cell. The chromosomes determine what characteristics a plant or animal will inherit.

CHRONIC. Lasting a long time. The opposite is *acute,* which refers to diseases that reach a crisis rapidly.

CLINICAL DISEASE. A disease advance enough that a doctor can recognize it from a patient's history and physical examination. (See also *subclinical disease.*)

COMBINATION CHEMOTHERAPY. Use of several different chemotherapeutic drugs at the same time.

CORTISONE. A hormone found in animals and often used to treat—among other things—inflammation, arthritis and allergies.

CURATIVE. Serving to cure or completely heal. (See also *palliative.*)

CYST. A fluid-filled sac that can be either benign or malignant.

DIAGNOSIS. Establishing the exact cause of an illness through examination; a doctor's opinion based on examination and investigation.

DNA (D-NUCLEIC ACID). Thread-shaped material in the nucleus of a cell that carries information about what will be inherited.

-ECTOMY. Word ending to indicate surgical removal of an organ (for example, tonsilectomy, appendectomy, or mastectomy).

EDEMA. An accumulation of fluids or a swelling.

ESTROGEN. A female hormone produced principally by ovaries in young women and by adrenal glands in older women.

ESTROGEN RECEPTORS. Proteins that carry estrogen and increase the ability of estrogen to function.

ETIOLOGY. The cause or origin of a disease.

EXCISION. Surgical removal of tissue.

EXPLORATORY SURGERY. Surgery performed to find the suspected cause of a problem.

GENES. Units in the body that determine what traits will be inherited.

GYNECOLOGY. The branch of medical science that deals with the diseases of women, especially those of the genital tract and the reproductive system.

HODGKIN'S DISEASE. A form of cancer of the lymph glands.

HORMONES. Chemicals formed in the body that regulate specific functions of the body.

IMMUNOLOGY. The study of the body's defense system against disease.

INFUSION. In medical usage, the introduction into a *vein* at a regulated rate. (See also perfusion.)

INTRA-ARTERIAL. Inside an artery.

INTRAMUSCULAR. Inside a muscle.

INTRAVENOUS. Inside a vein.

LESION. A wound, injury or abnormal body tissue.

LEUKEMIA. Any of several diseases involving uncontrolled proliferation of blood cells—usually white cells but occasionally red cells or platelets.

LINEAR ACCELERATOR. A highly accurate instrument used in radiation therapy to direct very high energy toward an organ.

LYMPH SYSTEM. A part of the circulatory system that collects body fluids and particles and either purifies or destroys the particles. It is a major part of the body's defense system.

LYMPH NODES. Tissues in the lymph system that destroy foreign or abnormal particles.

LYMPHOMA. Cancer of the lymph system.

MALIGNANT. Cancerous.

MAMMOGRAM. An X ray of the breast.

MASTECTOMY. Surgical removal of a breast and, in some cases, of nearby tissue.

MEGAVOLTAGE. High-energy radiation measured in millions of volts. The newest X-ray equipment produces energy in megavolts, which can be directed more precisely and with less risk of burns than the orthovoltage used in older equipment.

METASTASIS. The spread of a cancer from its original site to other organs.

MONITOR. To watch closely.

MYELOMA. Bone cancer.

NEUTRON-BEAM RADIATION. A new radiation technique that is effective against radioresistant cells.

-OMA. A tumor (for example, lymphoma or myeloma).

ONCOLOGY. The study of the diagnosis and treatment of cancer.

ONCOLOGIST. A specialist in the treatment of cancer.

ORAL. By mouth.

ORTHOVOLTAGE. Low-energy radiation measured in thousands of volts or kilovolts and produced by early X-ray equipment. Orthovoltage does not penetrate tissue as effectively as the new megavoltage equipment.

-OSTOMY. Word ending to indicate surgical construction of an artificial part (for example, colostomy is the construction of an artificial opening from the colon).

PALLIATIVE. Treatment aimed at relieving unpleasant symptoms when cure is unlikely.

PERFUSION. In medical terms, the injection of medication into the artery.

PLATELETS. Tiny blood cells responsible for preventing bleeding.

PROGNOSIS. A prediction of the likely outcome of an illness.

RADIATION THERAPY. A treatment in which minute high-energy particles bombard cancer cells to damage or destroy them.

RADIORESISTANT TUMORS. Tumors that require very large doses of radiation to damage them.

RADIOSENSITIVE TUMORS. Tumors that require only small doses of radiation to destroy them.

RAD. The unit of measuring the dose of radiation.

RED BLOOD CELLS. The blood cells that carry oxygen.

REMISSION. A tumor *in remission* is one that has shrunk in size or disappeared completely. Remission may be temporary; a tumor may reappear and resume growing.

SARCOMA. A cancer of connective tissues (such as muscles and fat cells) and some types of bone cancer.

SCAN. A special X ray that makes use of the fact that certain chemicals tend to concentrate in specific organs. In some illnesses, certain areas will absorb too much or too little of the chemicals, and a doctor looking at a scan (which looks like a photograph) may be able to estimate the extent of the illness.

SEMINOMA. A form of tumor of the testicle.

STABILIZATION. Stabilization of a tumor means that it is neither spreading nor shrinking.

STAGING. Determining the extent to which a tumor has spread.

SUBCLINICAL DISEASE. A disease in such an early stage that it cannot be detected through a patient's history and physical examination alone.

SUPPOSITORY. Medication given via the rectum.

TUMOR. An abnormal growth in the body. *(Tumor* and *cancer* are used interchangeably in this book.)

ULTRASONIC X RAY. An X ray that makes images by sending out sound waves. A patient does not receive radiation when an ultrasonic X ray is made.

VEIN. A blood vessel that returns blood *toward* the heart and lungs for purification. (See also *artery*.)

VENOUS. Having to do with the veins.

VIRUS. A disease-causing agent that can reproduce itself only when inside a living cell.

WHITE BLOOD CELLS. The bloods cells that fight infection.

Bibliography

CHAPTER ONE

DeVita, V.T., Jr. "Ten Years of Cancer Progress 1971–1981." *Cancer News* 36 (Winter, 1982): 4–5.
Einhorn, L.H., ed. *Testicular Tumors: Management and Treatment.* New York: Masson Publishing U.S.A., 1980.

CHAPTER TWO

Anderson, W.A.D. *Synopsis of Pathology.* 6th ed. St. Louis: C.V. Mosby, Co., 1964.
Bondeson, Lennart, et al. "Occult Thyroid Carcinoma at Autopsy in Malmo, Sweden." *Cancer* 47 (January 15, 1981): 319–23.
International Union against Cancer. *Illustrated Tumor Nomenclature.* 2nd ed. Berlin and New York: Springer-Verlag, 1969.
Ziegler, John L. "Management of Burkitt's Lymphoma: An Update." *Cancer Treatment Reviews* 6 (June, 1979): 95–105.

CHAPTER THREE

Ewing, James. Proceedings of the American Society for the Control of Cancer. New York: April, 1929.

CHAPTER FOUR

Arnott, S.J. "Advances in Radiotherapy." *Practitioner* 221 (October, 1978): 563–69.

Cattell, A. "Radiation—Discovery and Developments." *Nursing Mirror* 152 (March 19, 1981): ii–iii.

Krakoff, I.H. "Cancer Chemotherapeutic Agents." *Ca—A Cancer Journal for Clinicians* 23 (July/August, 1973): 209–19.

———"Cancer Chemotherapeutic Agents." *Ca—A Cancer Journal for Clinicians* 27 (May/June, 1977): 130–43.

Phillips, T.L. "Principles of Radiobiology and Radiation Therapy." In *Principles of Cancer Treatment*, edited by S.K. Carter, pp. 58–87. New York: McGraw-Hill, 1982.

Suit, H.D., et al. "Preoperative Radiation Therapy for Sarcoma of Soft Tissue." *Cancer* 47 (May 1, 1981): 2269–74.

Yarbro, J.W. "Future Prospects in Radiation Therapy." *Seminars in Oncology* 8 (March 1981).

CHAPTER SIX

Bakemeier, R.F. "Principles of Medical Oncology and Cancer Chemotherapy." In *Clinical Oncology for Medical Students and Physicians*, 5th ed., edited by P. Rubin, pp. 42–50. Rochester, N.Y.: University of Rochester, 1978.

Roffman, Roger. *Marijuana As Medicine.* Seattle: Madrona Publishers, 1982.

Rosner, Fred. "Is Chemotherapy Carcinogenic?" *Ca—A Cancer Journal for Clinicians* 28 (January/February, 1978): 57–59.

Seigel, L.J., et al. "The Control of Chemotherapy-Induced Emesis." *Annals of Internal Medicine* 95 (September, 1981): 352–59.

CHAPTER SEVEN

"Adjuvant Treatment of Colon Cancer. Results of a Prospectively Randomized Trial. Gastrointestinal Tumor Study Group." *New England Journal of Medicine* 310 (March 22, 1984): 737–43.

Axtell, L.M., ed. *Recent Trends in Survival of Cancer Patients, 1960–1971* (Supplement to End Results in Cancer; Report #4). Bethesda, Md., 1974.

Barber, H.R.K. "Ovarian Cancer. Part I." *Ca—A Cancer Journal for Clinicians* 29 (November/December, 1979): 341–51.

———"Ovarian Cancer. Part II." *Ca—A Cancer Journal for Clinicians* 30 (January/February, 1980): 2–15.

Burkitt, Dennis. "Etiology and Prevention of Colorectal Cancer." *Hospital Practice* 19 (February, 1984): 67–77.

Carbone, P.P. "Changing Strategy of Curative Treatment of Breast Cancer." In *Breast Cancer: Trends in Research and Treatment,* edited by J.C. Heuson, pp. 229–38. New York: Raven Press, 1976.

Carter, Stephen. *Principles of Cancer Treatment.* New York: McGraw-Hill, 1982.

Coltman, C.A., Jr. "Chemotherapy of Advanced Hodgkin's Disease." *Seminars in Oncology* 7 (June, 1980): 155–73.

Comis, R.L. "Therapy of Small-Cell Anaplastic Lung Cancer." *Clinical Cancer Briefs* (March, 1981): 3–11.

DeVita, V.T., Jr., et al. "Curability of Advanced Hodgkin's Disease with Chemotherapy." *Annals of Internal Medicine* 92 (May, 1980): 587–95.

Einhorn, L. H., et al. "Combination Chemotherapy in Disseminated Testicular Cancer: The Indiana University Experience." *Seminars in Oncology* 6 (March, 1979): 87–93.

———"The Management of Disseminated Testicular Cancer." In *Testicular Tumors: Management and Treatment,* edited by L.H. Einhorn, pp. 117–49. New York: Masson Publishing U.S.A., 1980.

Ginsberg, S.J., et al. "Long-Term Survivorship in Small-Cell Anaplastic Lung Carcinoma." *Cancer Treatment Reports* 63 (August, 1979): 1347–49.

Greco, F. Anthony, et al. *Gastrointestinal Cancer.* Pamphlet. Bristol Laboratories: Chicago, 1980.

Griffiths, C. T. "Gynecological Cancer" in *Cancer Medicine,* J. F. Holland, editor. Philadelphia: Lea & Febiger, 1973.

Jacobs, E.M., et al. "Testicular Cancer: Risk Factors and the Role of Adjuvant Chemotherapy." *Cancer* 45 (Suppl. 7, April 15, 1980): 1782–90.

———"Chemotherapy of Testicular Cancer: From Palliation to Curative Adjuvant Therapy." *Seminars in Oncology* 6 (March, 1979): 3–13.

Jacquillat, C., et al. "Combination Therapy in 130 Patients with Acute Lymphoblastic Leukemia (Protocol 06 LA 66-Paris)." *Cancer Research* 33 (December, 1973): 3278–84.

Livingston, R.B. "Treatment of Small-Cell Carcinoma: Evolution and Future Directions." *Seminars in Oncology* 5 (September, 1978): 299–308.

Marchant, D.J. "Ovarian Carcinoma: Staging and Surgical Treatment." *Current Concepts in Oncology* (July/August, 1981): 3–11.

Mauer, A.M. "Treatment of Acute Leukemia in Children." *Clinics in Hematology* 7 (June, 1978): 245–58.

135

Mauer, A.M., et al. "The Current Status of the Treatment of Child-hood Acute Lymphoblastic Leukemia." *Cancer Treatment Reviews* 3 (March, 1976): 17–41.

Martini, N., et al. "Oat Cell Carcinoma of the Lung." *Clinical Bulletin* 5 (1975): 144–48.

Seydel, H. Gunter, et al. "Radiation Therapy in Small Cell Lung Cancer." *Seminars in Oncology* 5 (September, 1978): 288–98.

Sherlock, Paul. "Colorectal Cancer: Expanding Role for the Family Physician." *Oncology News* (July, 1982).

Vincent, R.G., et al. "Progress in the Chemotherapy of Small Cell Carcinoma of the Lung." *Cancer* 47 (January 15, 1981): 229–35.

Woodruff, R. "The Management of Adult Acute Lymphoblastic Leukemia." *Cancer Treatment Reviews* 5 (June, 1978): 95–113.

CHAPTER NINE

Aledort, L.M. "AIDS: An Update." *Hospital Practice* 18 (September, 1983): 159.

Burkhardt, S.S. "The Medical Use of Lasers." *Journal of the Operating Room Research Institute* 2 (April, 1982): 10–21.

Cattell, A. "Radiation—Discovery and Developments." *Nursing Mirror* 152 (March 19, 1981): ii–iii.

Dixon, J.A. "Surgical Applications of Lasers." *Bulletin of the American College of Surgeons* 67 (November, 1982): 4–9.

Foster, C. S. "Lymphocyte Hybridomas." *Cancer Treatment Reviews* 9 (June, 1982): 59–84.

Insel, R.A., et al. "Monoclonal Antibodies: Clinical Relevance to Pediatrics." *American Journal of Diseases of Children* 137 (January, 1983): 69–76.

Jaffe, H.W., et al. "National Case-Control Study of Kaposi's Sarcoma and *Pneumocystis carinii* Pneumonia in Homosexual Men: Part 1, Epidemiologic Results." *Annals of Internal Medicine*, 99 (August, 1983): 145–51.

Milstein, C. "Monoclonal Antibodies." *Cancer*, 49 (May 15, 1982): 1953–57.

Priestman, T.J. "Interferon: An Anti-Cancer Agent?" *Cancer Treatment Reviews* 6 (December, 1979): 223–37.

Ziegler, John L. "Management of Burkitt's Lymphoma: An Update." *Cancer Treatment Reviews* 6 (June, 1979) 95–105.

Zubrod, C. Gordon. "Historic Milestones in Curative Chemotherapy." *Seminars in Oncology* 6 (December, 1979): 490–505

APPENDIX: A Guide to Chemotherapeutic Drugs

Bakemeier, R.F. "Principles of Medical Oncology and Cancer Chemotherapy." In *Clinical Oncology for Medical Students and Physicians*, 5th ed., edited by P. Rubin, pp. 42–50. Rochester: University of Rochester, 1978.

Greenwald, E.S. *Cancer Chemotherapy*, 2nd ed., Flushing, N.Y.: Medical Examination Publishing Co., 1982.

Holland, J.F., ed. *Cancer Medicine.* Philadelphia: Lea & Febiger, 1973.

Issell, B.F., et al. "Etoposide (VP–16–213)." *Cancer Treatment Reviews* 6 (June, 1979): 107–24.

Krakoff, I.H. "Cancer Chemotherapeutic Agents." *Ca—A Cancer Journal for Clinicians* 23 (July/August, 1973): 209–19.

———"Cancer Chemotherapeutic Agents." *Ca—A Cancer Journal for Clinicians* 27 (May/June, 1977): 130–43.

Index